The Business of Chiropractic: How To Prosper After Startup

I would highly recommend this book for any professional starting or continuing in a business...The management concepts provided are well presented and easily adaptable. Additionally, although professionals would agree with the ideas set forth in the book, we forget to implement them and it is an enjoyable way to be reminded.

Marsha K. Niedens
Attorney-at-law, Camarillo, California

I just read your book and I wish I had read it long ago. It would have saved me a lot of time and money over the last several years....I heartily recommend it to any established or new DC. I have seen nothing like it before.

Richard E. Rogovin, D.C.
Valrico, Florida

This book synthesizes the most difficult subject of Business Management into a concise and easily readable form which will undoubtedly stand as the definitive work in this area of Chiropractic practice.

Thomas V. Giordano, D.C.
LECCE, Italia

Great, realistic and effective ideas on running a successful practice. It includes everything from marketing to internal management with real life experiences.

Michael D. Beattie, D.C.
Waterloo Chiropractic Health Centre, Canada

The Business Of Chiropractic *is an easy-to-read how-to book. Field practitioners will learn personal, professional and business methods which can lead to a prosperous practice.*
  It is truly a blueprint for success.

Moses Jacob, D.C.
Novato Chiropractic Office, Novato, California

This book is recommended for new Chiropractors and practicing D.C.'s alike. The information about business ideas and plans is a must for the successful Chiropractor / Businessman.

Bert Vanderbliek, D.C.
A Chiropractic Group
Reseda, California

I have just finished your excellent book on chiropractic management and I must say I was delighted. It is a common sense approach to every situation the individual doctor will encounter with just the right amount of humor mixed in. I found myself smiling while making margin notes on some "gem" I had found in the text....

Douglas R. Guyot, D.C.
Guyot Chiropractic
Sevierville, Tennessee

Many books and publications have delineated the application and practice of chiropractic as a natural healing art. A number of vantage points of the chiropractic profession abound which are available in bookstores, seminars, colleges, and by direct order.

Although many publications serve well the needs of chiropractic practice, the approach of Dr. Ivan Delman will truly fulfill a special niche. After earning the bachelor of science in business administration degree at Roosevelt University in Chicago, Ivan Delman then graduated from Cleveland College, Los Angeles Campus, with the doctor of chiropractic degree. To bring the "virtual" reality of a practice spanning almost two decades, and merge business administration principles throughout the evolutionary growth of the ensuing service business, gives chiropractic a forceful reality that has previously been minimized.

This step-by-step approach to chiropractic practice with the direct business overlay will be most helpful to graduates initiating an office. Furthermore, those practitioners already in established practices will find the business administration approach invaluable in the present day competitive marketplace.

From the "Foreword" to the first edition, by Edwin D. Follick, Dean and Chaplain, Cleveland Chiropractic College, Los Angeles, California

The **Business** Of Chiropractic

How to Prosper *after* Startup

Second Edition

Ivan Delman, D.C.

Business of Chiropractic
Dandridge, Tennessee

The Business of Chiropractic: How To Prosper After Startup, Second Edition

Notice to the Reader: This book is intended to provide information in regard to the subject matter covered. It is sold with the understanding that the publisher and author are not engaged in rendering legal, accounting, or similar services. If legal or other expert assistance is required, the services of a competent professional should be sought.

Every effort has been made to make this book as complete and as accurate as possible. However, there may be mistakes in both typography and content. This text should be used only as a general guide and not as the ultimate source of practice management information. Furthermore, this book contains information on practice management accurate only up to the printing date.

The purpose of this book is to educate in an entertaining manner. The author and Business of Chiropractic Publications shall have neither liability nor responsibility to any person or entity with respect to any loss or damage caused, or alleged to be caused, directly or indirectly by the information contained in this book.

If you do not wish to be bound by the above, you may return this book to the publisher for a full refund.

Copyright © 1999, 2002 by Ivan Delman. All rights reserved. This work may not be copied, stored, reproduced, retrieved, or transmitted by any means whatsoever without prior, written permission of the author, except for brief passages quoted in review. For information, contact Business of Chiropractic Publications, 1227 Cedar Hill Road, Dandridge, TN 37725 <http://www.businessofchiropractic.com>.

Text and cover design by Robert Goodman, Silvercat®, San Diego, California

Second printing, August, 2002

ISBN 0-9669892-1-X

Publishers Cataloging-in-Publication Data
(Provided by Quality Books, Inc.)

Delman, Ivan.
   The business of chiropractic : how to prosper after
  startup / Ivan Delman – 2nd ed.
    p. cm.
   ISBN: 0-9669892-1-X

     1. Chiropractic–Practice.   2. Chiropractic offices--
Management.   I. Title.

   RZ232.2.D25 2002   615.5'34'068
                                      QBI02-200285

Printed in the United States of America

This book is dedicated to the memory of my mother, Melva.

Mom, thank you for leaving me your gypsy passion. It's brightened the colors of my life.

You're in my heart.

Contents

***Second Edition Foreword*, by Robert L. Dubin, DC** .... *xi*
Preface: The Genesis Of This Book .... *xiii*
    Why This Book? .... *xiv*
    Acknowledgments .... *xv*

1 Where Does Your Money Go? 17
    Think Management 17
    Why Managers And Race Car Drivers Are Kindred 17
    A Positive Attitude Achieves Success 18
    Start Learning the Business of Your Business 19
    Shared Traits of Successful Managers 20
    What Does A Manager Do? 22

2 Four Essential Clinic Functions 25
    Basic Planning 25
    Personnel 26
    Operations 29
    Finances 29

3 Powerful Ethics: The Keystone Of A Strong Practice 31

4 Four Easy Steps To Decision-Making 33
    Some Tips To Help You Avoid Procrastinating 34
    Let It Go! 35

5 How To Delegate Rather Than Relegate 37
    Try This Example 37

6 Prioritize Before You Decide 39
    List Your Priorities 39

7	*Practice Basics Worth Repeating* 43
	The Basics 44
8	*Free Advice: Worth What You Pay For It* 49
9	*Why You Need A Mission Statement* 51
	A Side Benefit 52
10	*How To Set Goals* 55
	How To Set Goals And Objectives? 57
11	*Blueprint For Success: Your Business Plan* 61
	Plan is not a four-letter word 61
	Five Easy Questions 62
	Delman Chiropractic Marketing Guide 65
12	*Duties Of A Practice Manager* 67
13	*Developing Yourself As A Manager* 71
	Pushing Your Limits 71
	Taking Risks 72
	D.A.R.E. to Risk 72
	Keeping Your Goals In Sight 74
	A Complacency Check 75
	Changing Procedures In Small Increments 76
	Methods That Will Advance Your Practice 76
	Take Care Of The Big Rocks First! 78
	Phone Interruptions 79
	Community Service 80
14	*How To Reduce Paperwork Time* 83
	You Don't Have to Write *War and Peace!* 83
	Stock Phrases And How To Find Them 83
	An Alternative Method 85
15	*Cash Flow* 87
	Profits and Cash Flow 87
	Cash-flow Projections 88
	Interpreting The Cash Flow Projection 89
	Why You Should Chart Statistics 91
	Start By Asking Questions 92
	Charting Practice Trends 92
	How To Build Your Charts 93
	Start With These Numbers 98
16	*Your Management Style* 99
	The Big Picture 99
	Get Off Your Duff and Manage! 99
	Looking for the Tip of the Iceberg 101
	Are You Listening? 102
	Do Your Patients Fall Asleep During the ROF? 103

  On Being Polite 103
  I'm Managing Everything! 104
  Bend or Break 104
  Teamwork or Tomahawk? 105
  Directing Your Staff 106
  We're Too Busy for New Patients? 106
  Working Hard versus Working Smart 107
  Alternative Plans Just in Case 108

17 *Diagnosing Your Practice By Priority* *111*

18 *Retaining Patients* *115*
  The Doctor/Patient Relationship 116
  Scratch That Niche! 116
  Watch Your Language 117
  Involve Your Patients 118
  Get Feedback 118

19 *Inventory Control* *121*
  Is Your Practice An Inventory Smithsonian? 121
  How to Reduce the Cost of Inventory 123
  Types Of Inventory 123

20 *Personnel Matters* *127*
  The Importance of Harmony 127
  Your Safety Belt: Your Staff 128
  Hey! Aunt Millie! Want a Job? 129
  Staff Meetings: Monologue or Dialogue? 131
  The Need To Know 132
  Policy Manuals 134
  Topics Covered in a Good Manual 135
  Evaluating Personnel 137

21 *Marketing* *139*
  I'm A Doctor, Not A Salesman! 139
  Marketing, Sales, Outreach, Whatever! 141
  Marketing a Service 141
  Your Position in the Community 142
  Determining the Market for Your Services 144

22 *Advertising* *149*
  To Advertise Or Not, That's The Question 149
  Successful Advertising Strategies 150
  Advertising Lessons We Have Learned 151
  A Secret Weapon: Your Business Card 154
  Writing Your Own Advertising Copy 155
  Other Types of Advertising 157
  A Final Advertising Thought 158

23	***On Looking As You Wish To Be***	*159*
24	***Lessons Others Have Taught Me***	*161*
	Choices	161
	Promote With Class	162
	Associate With Winners	163
	Ethics Do Matter	163
	Showcase Your Talent	164
	A Synergistic Suggestion	164
25	***Making It All Work***	*165*
	Finding out what works	166
	Decision-Making Made Easy	167
	Why You Need An Information Partner	168
	Only Use What's Comfortable	170
	Rubber Walls For Your Goals	171
	The Importance Of You In Your Practice	172
26	***A Short Recap***	*175*
Sources, Resources, And Recommended Reading		*177*

Second Edition Foreword

Dr. Delman has done what seemed impossible - he has actually improved upon his earlier work, by adding 20% new material, 11 new and stimulating articles, and 4 brand new chapters, including a broad overview of the process of making a Chiropractic office work for the Doctor.

The second edition of The Business of Chiropractic is more comprehensive, more entertaining, more specific and focused - in short, it is a great improvement on an already superb product.

From A to Z, Dr. Delman guides the reader through the painstaking process of creating a successful business and serving humanity simultaneously, and he does it with humor and with well reasoned and tried and true marketing methods, which at once illuminate the subject and present it in a very palatable format which the reader can immediately implement to his or her benefit.

I am especially struck by the comprehensive listing of sources, recommended reading and resources at the end of the book, which is quite complete, and which contains references to the best sources of such information in existence.

This resource list alone makes the price of the book an incredible bargain.

Overall, Dr. Delman has done a real service to his profession once again, by combining his educational and professional experience into this step by step guide for his fellow practitioners, who, if they follow his impeccable instructions, can't help but succeed in practice.

Thanks, Ivan, you are a real asset to Chiropractic!

Robert L. Dubin, DC
President,
California Chiropractic Association (2000 - 2002)

*Give a man a fish and you feed him for a day.
Teach him to fish and you feed him for a lifetime.*
—Chinese Proverb.

Preface:
The Genesis Of This Book

Good Grief! Another book on practice management? Hold on! This is different! This book will give you step-by-step directions on how to follow the road to having an enjoyable, prosperous practice. Have the other books accomplished this for you?

Follow me as I traveled the road to this book.

In 1959, I graduated from college with a degree in business. For the next twenty years, my career path was focused on the management of manufacturing plants then claims management in the insurance industry. While investigating claims involving chiropractic care, I gradually realized it was a profession that made sense and contributed positively to the health of the community. So rather than be an opponent of chiropractors, I decided to become one.

I obtained my California DC license in 1978 and immediately opened my own clinic. There were eventually five facilities. However, my eventual preference was a single clinic. During my seventeen-plus years in practice, business management never seemed to be a serious problem since practice operations utilized standard business principles. From 1978 until my retirement in 1995, my operating statistics were positive regardless of the state of the economy.

I saw from 200 to 250 patients per week working three full days and two half days with no weekends. During the 90s, our gross income varied between $550,000 to $600,000 with relatively low overhead. Our net profit averaged between 50 and 60 percent.

I thought most experienced solo practitioners produced about the same numbers. I was wrong!

After an accident prompted retirement, my wife and I packed up and traveled around the USA. Whenever possible, we would go to a local DC for an adjustment and get together. During our visits, I discovered too many chiropractors, although competent in their craft, were having difficulty operating their clinics profitably. I realized the doctors struggling with the survival of their practice were unaware of basic business principles.

When discussing business matters, I noticed that, regardless of their location in this country, the chiropractor's questions addressed a common subject: the business aspects of operating a chiropractic practice. After we discussed their particular business problems, I outlined some basic business plans designed to get their practices growing and prospering.

Follow up discussions with the doctors indicated their clinics were now easier to manage and profits were on the increase as a result of their applying basic business principles to their practice.

Based upon our three years of field consulting, it's obvious that there's a business crisis developing in many chiropractic practices. The doctor, although competent in his craft, is trying to operate his business with insufficient information on how to do it properly. That doctor needs information! This book will provide that information.

Why This Book? I know that illustrating essential practice management concepts in a concise, uncomplicated manner can save hours of research for a busy doctor.

There are thousands of good books on management and business operating principles. Who has time to read all of them? This book saves time by gathering then presenting fundamental business concepts and their applications. All you have to do is put them to work!

This book was written with you, the busy doctor, in mind. It contains no-nonsense, useable information on how to successfully manage your office. Concepts which were tried and proven successful over more than seventeen years in active practice.

A chiropractic office functions the same as any other small business. Your office can be divided into basic operating groups. Once you understand the operational role these groups perform, you will discover the how easy it is to manage your office.

There are chapters in my book which show you how to:

- Apply an easy system for setting measurable goals using examples.
- How to solve your problems by developing, then prioritizing, your decision-making processes.
- Build an office staff you can lean on utilizing mobile management and other basic personnel methods.
- Establish harmony in your practice allowing it to grow and prosper.
- Use five proven concepts to guide your advertising programs.
- Write your own copy using eight tried and tested rules.
- Utilize office statistics in making sound management decisions for your clinic by following my simple guidelines.
- Make and utilize charts that will give you advance notice of problems affecting the future of your practice.

The information contained in my book will give you an insider's view on how to successfully maintain practice growth in your community regardless of current economic conditions. This information will alter your perceptions and provide you the needed facts necessary for sound management decisions.

Join the select group of doctors who consistently examine their clinic operations using these types of questions:

- What areas of my practice do I have to strengthen?
- What strategic planning will I have to formulate to be competitive in the changing marketplace?
- What changes in my practice will I have to make to keep it growing and being profitable?

If the above questions intrigue you, I urge you to read my book. It will give you the answers we discovered resulting in sustained practice growth for more than seventeen years.

It is not the purpose of this book to reprint all the information that is otherwise available to the author and/or the publisher, but to complement, amplify, and supplement other texts. You are urged to read all the available material, learn as much as possible about practice management and tailor the information to your individual needs. For more information, see the many references in the *Sources, Resources, and Recommended Reading* section.

Practice management requires the same intelligence, effort and creativity as patient care. It is not a get-rich-quick situation. The rewards are as much emotional as financial. Those who have been successful are aware of that fact. Those who will be successful are in for a pleasant experience.

This book is intended to be used, not just read. Use a highlighter. Dog-ear the pages. Take notes in the wide margins. I'll feel very satisfied if this book becomes the most shopworn book in your library. The essential components for a successful practice are at your fingertips. Check them out. Put them to work. Make them part of your practice. If you let them, they can help you turn the corner to a successful, rewarding chiropractic practice.

Acknowledgments

Over the two and a half years this book was coming together, I have been helped by so many people, it would take another book to list their names. I'll try to name a very few; to those whom I've not named, please know you have my sincere gratitude for your help.

The first person with the courage to read and edit my rambling manuscript was my brother Owen. He's a retired English professor, successful playwright, scriptwriter, and entrepreneur. He ran out of red ink on the first go-around, but he stuck with it and his suggestions (sometimes not so brotherly) formed the basis for a more cogent manuscript.

To the many chiropractors who have generously reviewed my rough drafts and taken the time to offer their helpful comments, I thank you.

To Gary Erkfritz, D.C. (An author in his own right) who gave thirty years to his profession for the betterment of his community, thanks for "loaning" me an afternoon and the book on publishing which started all this.

To my Internet pals on the chiropractic and publishing lists, thank you for your ideas and comments.

To Robert Goodman (Silvercat Publications) who designed the cover and text, thanks for not screaming when I asked the same question three times.

To my father, Philip Delman, one of the most common-sense people I have ever known. A successful businessman who, in his ninth decade, continues to challenge his mind with continued business activities. He has been and fortunately continues to be a valuable resource. He has taught me how making logical decisions will result in living life to its fullest. Thanks, Dad.

Of course, to my wife, Arlene who patiently listened to my prattlings, taped important car races and who provided the space, time, and encouragement to finish this project...my love and gratitude!

1

Where Does Your Money Go?

It's the first of the month. You enter your office half an hour before your first patient and start paying bills. As usual, you don't have enough in the bank to pay them all, so you start performing a "Barnum and Bailey" (a juggling act to determine which bills get paid and which don't).

Don't go through this trauma every month! You can succeed and prosper by hitching a ride on a winning attitude. But your chances are a lot better if you have the right management frame of mind.

Think Management

The wisest mind has something yet to learn.
—George Santayana

You've already been through the shock-reality of practice start-up and have been operating for several years. You have enough patients to keep you busy. Yet, you still are unstable; money, time, and pleasure continue to be in short supply.

Your practice is on a plateau: no matter how hard you work, results continue to be less than expectations. You are struggling because the business of chiropractic is low on your priority list. Think of yourself not just as a chiropractor, but also as a business owner.

Why Managers And Race Car Drivers Are Kindred

Managers and race car drivers have much in common. They both had to learn their trade prior to being competitive in their endeavors.

Race car drivers and other competitive types vary in their performances. They all learn the same rules, tricks, techniques, and so on. However, some have better reaction times, some are in better shape, and some can think more clearly behind the wheel. Those traits, many times, are innate. But they still have to learn the "the game" (whatever that might be) before they can start to excel at their craft.

Managers are in the same boat. They may have some people skills. They may be "quick on their feet." But they will have to *learn* to be good managers. Managing a practice is a learned skill. When you learn to manage and then combine that knowledge with a winning attitude, you position yourself to achieve success.

A Positive Attitude Achieves Success

Your attitude, not your aptitude will determine your altitude.
—Zig Zeigler

Applying a positive attitude to basic fundamentals will make you a winner.

The person with a negative attitude who expects to fail will succeed in failing. For example, have you ever walked across an open grating holding a set of keys? You kept telling yourself, "Don't drop the keys. Don't drop the keys." How close did you come to dropping them? Have you ever stood on the edge of a cliff, looking down saying, "I don't want to fall. I don't want to fall"? Then you felt yourself leaning closer to the edge. That's thinking like a loser!

The old saw that says, "You'll reap what you sow," holds true for attitude. If you plant a success attitude, you'll harvest what you planted. The opposite also holds true.

The successful doctor has a success-oriented perspective. He or she has "attitude"!

A competitor on a winning streak sustains a winning attitude. One win feeds the next. Fifty percent of the winning equation is attitude; this productive streak will continue until the winning equation is lost.

Most successful people are competitive with themselves. Instead of wasting their time and energy looking in the rear view mirror, they constantly strive to improve.

When I was still in practice, a newspaper reporter asked me about several new chiropractors who just opened up in our town. The reporter's question was, "Does all the new competition affect your practice?" My answer was, "Not at all! My only competition is myself." That's a positive attitude!

If you look around at business friends in trouble, their problems are usually caused by themselves, not some outside source. Sure, business climates change. However, you are responsible for being aware and changing your operations to fit the situation. An example of a changing situation is the health care market. There are many more groups now vying for the same piece of the health care market. Operating your practice and ignoring the changes is an accident waiting to happen. No matter what your colleagues are doing, you must make changes or shortly you'll suffer the consequences of your inactions.

Remember, if you affiliate with people who have losing attitudes, you'll *also* start thinking like a loser. If you want to be successful, find people who are already successful and associate with them. They expect to win, and they do win more often than they lose. When people are successful over a sustained period, it becomes ingrained in their thinking. For them, the second place finisher is just the first loser. For them, anything but success is unthinkable!

(A comment on the word, *success*. Everyone has his or her own view of what they perceive to be success. To me, success means achieving my goals, whether they are philosophical or material; however, when you see the word "success," just insert your own definition of that term.)

Start Learning the Business of Your Business

You've hammered away at school, passed your boards, and now you're a Doctor of Chiropractic.

You've made the courageous decision to have your own office. You put together all the initial components for your practice. You are a knowledgeable, ethical doctor. You survived the startup. You now are bumping along the solo practitioner's road. You are still encumbered with debts. It seems no matter how hard you work, your business dwells on an unchanging plateau.

Does that sound like your present situation?

Where do you go from here? You know you are a good Doctor of Chiropractic, but how much do you know about the business of running your business?

Nature does not tolerate stasis. You must be certain you are moving forward with your business as well as your chiropractic plans.

If your experience was like mine, the business courses you attended in chiropractic college were thin in content, not related to the real world, and even, at times, insulting to your intelligence.

I remember one "instructor" in a business class. He was a typical side-stepper. When asked a question for which he had no answer, he'd say, "We'll get to that later." Of course, we never did.

At semester's end, we left him a message on the blackboard, "Now is later!"

Chiropractic colleges state that their business is to educate chiropractors. Unfortunately, too many do not feel their duty includes helping provide those chiropractors with the skills necessary to survive in today's business world!

Chiropractic colleges historically have relegated business training to a few perfunctory in-house classes. I sincerely hope that sad situation improves. Knowledge of the basic business essentials are a necessity for a person to successfully run his own clinic.

If you were lucky, your business instructor had been successful in his clinic operations and was willing to share his experiences. He will have offered his opinion on how to:

- Develop your management skills
- Develop the tools that can demonstrate past, present and future clinic trends
- Utilize successful advertising strategies
- Determine whether or not you want to be involved with associates
- Mold your practice and staff into a successful, synergistic, goal-oriented unit.

Unless you've been actively working on the above concepts, it's time to start because, "Now Is Later!"

Shared Traits of Successful Managers

Successful people in business share similar traits, no matter the businesses in which they are involved. Working hard, by itself, does not guarantee success. Don't confuse activity with achievement! Activity with satisfying results leaves me less tired at the end of the day than the same activity with limited results. Your activity must include other elements in order to accomplish results. Having a mission (purpose) and striving for results are important parts of a successful program. The people who "Get things done" know how to assemble all the elements of a winning program.

Let's look at some characteristics of people who are able to put together the essential elements leading to successful operations and see how you match up.

On the facing page is a test that encompasses some of their basic attributes. Take the test now. Circle the answer which most closely relates to you.

If you circled yes to the majority of the questions, you possess many successful business personality traits. Your no answers point to areas that need your attention. Bolstering a weak area is far more important than further strengthening one already strong. Your management skills must be as solid as your business

Successful Manager Self Test

Self-Control

   Do you:

Y N Feel uncomfortable in structured environments such as school?
Y N Perceive you are superior to the majority of your peers?
Y N Sense you are superior to the majority of your superiors?
Y N Have an uneasy feeling with someone having authority over you?
Y N Enjoy creating methods and tactics to overcome problems?
Y N Need freedom to determine then proceed taking action on your own perceptions?

Comprehensive Awareness

   Do you:

Y N Plan several steps ahead as you travel your business road?
Y N Constantly watch the important details of your business?
Y N Make operational decisions based on your business objectives?

Sense Of Urgency

   Do you:

Y N Prefer energetic activities while on vacation?
Y N Feel a sense of urgency in your lifestyle?
Y N Prefer individual over team sports?
Y N Pursue your goals with a high level of energy?

Realism

   Are you:

Y N Pragmatic in your assessment of a situation?
Y N Willing to change direction after making a decision?
Y N Frequently reviewing the status of any given situation?
Y N In the habit of verifying information to determine its veracity?

Interpersonal Relationships

   Are you:

Y N More concerned with people's accomplishments than their feelings?
Y N Able to sever relationships which endanger your business?
Y N Driving your employees as hard as you push yourself?

This points to a traditional style of business success: the driven, achieving entrepreneur. This is the model I come from, and since I write out of my own experience, to some extent, this book reflects my prejudice toward the "type A" way of doing things.

Yet, I recognize that other approaches may be valid. Many chiropractors are driven first and foremost by their desire to heal, to make a difference in people's lives. If you are this style of chiropractor, you may or may not have a lot of the traditional entrepreneurial skills and styles. If so, you'll need to adapt the techniques in this book to your own personal style: to find ways of running your office that feel appropriate to your practice. You still share goals with the more entrepreneurial-driven practices. Your shared goals are to:

- Have enough free time in your work week to enjoy the things that make life worth living.
- Achieve enough financial success to live comfortably, pay all your office expenses, and have enough left over to finance both your present interests and your eventual retirement.
- Create a practice where the flow of patients is efficient, where you can help the greatest number of patients without feeling overwhelmed or overworked.

If the concepts of running your practice as a profit-driven business feel alien to you, I urge you to acknowledge your hesitation, recognize your own motivations, and understand that even the most patient-centered practice still needs to run as a profitable business. You can take the principles we discuss in these pages and work out models for those principles in a practice that has your own personal style all over it. But, if you neglect these principles entirely, you set yourself up for failure. Take what is useful, and think about the rest of it.

What Does A Manager Do?

Sometimes a manger will make money by ability, but usually by mistake.
—Business Proverb

Delineating the basic duties of a manager is not easy. Don't be tricked into thinking that having your business plan, opening your office, and printing your stationary is the beginning of your management experience. It's not! Management starts at the very beginning; when you take your first business breath. It continues as you get involved in the complexities of many personalities, the daily variables of practice operations, and the constant monitoring of always-changing goals. These concepts were not presented during my studies in chiropractic college.

If you are like most chiropractors, you don't have a management background. You find it easier to be involved in what you do best: treating your patients. Whether it's by omission or commission, management of your clinic may now be handled by someone else. If this is the case, your practice might be currently managed by a person who has a different mission. If you want to own and run a successful practice then it must be managed by you. It's that simple!

Having the loudest voice doesn't mean you're management material. You get in control when you decide to lead, then to manage. When one leads, they create criteria and directions. When one manages, those criteria and directions are guided and coordinated. A manager must perform both functions.

Your decision to become a strong manager is an essential element of your office operations. You set, then enforce, the way you want to run your show.

Despite your well thought-out decisions, you're still going to make mistakes. As long as you recognize a mistake and don't repeat it again, you'll make progress. If your successful decisions outweigh your failures, you'll move forward. As you work on your managing skills, your mistakes will decrease. The learning never stops. Reading the pertinent literature and attending the applicable seminars will maintain your business skills as you progress in your career. As in nature, there is no stasis.

2

Four Essential Clinic Functions

The Small Business Administration (SBA) performed studies of 900 small business operations to determine what the small business owner/manager needed to successfully function. One of the purposes of these studies was to figure out causes for the sixty-three percent failure rate of small business operations within their first six years. The results revealed four critical areas an owner must manage in order to survive: Basic Planning, Personnel, Operations, and Finances.

You might think the above is so obvious that I'm one neuron short of a synapse to mention it. These areas were not obvious to the owners of those whose business failed.

Let's look at those four areas and their components:

Basic Planning   Basic Planning is an area many practitioners overlook. Many doctors do not feel it is necessary to put their plans in writing. They feel planning will happen by "just keeping those plans in mind." This doesn't work. The operating details of your practice will obliterate those "thoughts" regarding basic planning. A written reference is essential to maintain your direction.

Your plan should include:

Mission Formulation. What is the reason for your practice's existence? The mission statement indicates why you exist and in what manner. For example, a mission statement could be, "I intend to better the health of local sports teams."

Marketing Plan Development. A marketing plan takes what you know about your patient base, analyzes its demographics, and develops an approach to that base. Marketing plans identify the services you want to offer and to whom. Once you decide on a particular segment of the market, you then plan how you will go about recruiting and serving it.

Fee Structure. To your patients, your fees are an important consideration. Fees form a picture in the patient's mind, accurate or not, about you and your practice. If they're noticeably lower or higher than your community then your practice is perceived as either low quality or too rich for their budget. In my experience, the future of chiropractic incomes is in cash practices, so I recommend setting fees that present the least resistance in your community.

There is no single fee that is the ideal. Instead, there is an acceptable range for your market. Survey the fees charged by other chiropractors in your community. Once you gather this data, select a reasonable fee structure that will be as easy as possible for a patient's budget. At the same time, your fees must take into account your operating expenses and desired profits.

A lower fee structure places added responsibility on the doctor/manager to:

- Minimize overhead costs (rent, unproductive equipment, salaries, loan payments, etc.)
- Place greater emphasis on patient education (back classes, a strong Report of Findings, creative use of educational pamphlets)
- Create a smooth, higher volume patient flow (tighter scheduling, the movement of patients within your office, the sequence of services you offer).

Create a Budget. This can be very complex or quite simple. Since your practice has been up and going for a while, you have data which you can use for your budgeting. For the simple budget, set percentage bases for salaries, advertising, purchasing, and promotion. The percentages can all be based on your gross income, then translated to monthly amounts.

If you have the time, you can keep the records. Otherwise, let your CPA supply the figures then you only have to manage the expenditures.

Personnel Planning for your personnel needs is necessary for a strong practice. The proportional losses are more acute in smaller offices.

You've lost half your total staff when one person of a two-person office is gone. The remaining employee's workload is now drastically increased until well after a new employee is trained. If you don't lose the overworked staff member, he or she will start to burn out and be less help to you. It's easier to keep good employees than train new ones especially if they can help you in the back room and at the front desk. Plan staffing for your growth as well as possible decline.

Planning for growth. While many offices have carefully laid plans for down-sizing their staff, fewer offices plan as carefully for growth. Give the same attention to both; they are equally important.

Consider local, part-time staffing before thinking of full timers:

- The benefit package for a part time employee is less or nonexistent
- There is greater flexibility in scheduling as well as cross training
- The need for extra staffing may be for only two or three days per week.
- They often require less time off for personal reasons
- As local residents, they will promote you to their neighbors.

Creating Job Descriptions. A doctor operating a small clinic might feel job descriptions are for the "Big Boys." Not true! As soon as you hire your first employee, you must have a way to tell your employee what is expected of her. That is your first reason for a job description. As you grow, job descriptions become even more critical as the lines become blurred between the various jobs in your clinic.

Developing a Job Description. Since you are already in operation, this will take a little more time than if you are first starting out in practice. Taking these simple steps now will avoid a lot of personnel friction later:

- Take a detailed look at all the jobs now being performed in your office.
- Write down all the facts pertaining to those jobs.
- Separate the various jobs into logical groups such as Front Desk, Insurance, Collections, and Back Room.
- Using the job descriptions as a guideline, write a profile of your future employee.

When you have completed this survey, you'll have information to help you make an informed decision when hiring as well as an outline of the duties and responsibilities of the job.

Hiring Staff. You are gambling against the odds if you think placing an ad or having one interview is going to produce the ideal employee. This may work for a manufacturing plant or grocery store, but it doesn't work in a chiropractic office.

There is an additional element you will want in an employee: that employee must have an interest in advancing the health of your patients.

By following these steps, you'll develop a staff of productive, long-term employees:

- Retrieve the appropriate job description you previously developed.
- Determine the profile you are seeking for this particular job.
- Place an ad advising the applicant to call during certain times. These will be the times you are available to talk to the applicant.
- When the applicant calls, pre-screen this prospect regarding acceptable hours, salary requirements, and requirements of the applicant. You can also inform the prospect of the job parameters in more detail than the ad did. This also gives you the opportunity to listen to the applicant. You'll be able to determine if they have speak clearly and have a "phone personality."
- Invite all the applicants who pass your pre-screening to a short meeting, during off-hours, as a group.
- The group meeting is the time to give all the applicants a shortened version of your New Patient Spinal Class seminar. Observe the applicants while you are speaking. Those who fall asleep should not be seriously considered!
- After the short meeting, provide refreshments. This will allow you to meet each person and observe the way they handle themselves with others. Making a choice will be easy after the meeting.

A Couple of additional reminders:

- When your new employee is hired, make up a training schedule and adhere to it.
- Assign your new hire to a member of your staff who is not leaving. A new hire trained by a leaving employee will not be as effective as one trained by more stable personnel.
- Don't pick the first applicant without looking at all the available choices.
- Don't choose an applicant just because time is running out. It is easier on the stability of your office to find temporary help, until you find the "Right" employee.

(Additional personnel subjects are discussed later in this book.)

Putting Together a Personnel Manual. Personnel protocols will use more of your time and energy than any other practice activity. How many times have you thought, "If I could only run this place myself!" Of course you can if you want to maintain a one-patient-per-hour-practice! Otherwise, your staff are essential to the survival and growth of your practice. A properly developed personnel manual is indispensable in employee relations.

I do not recommend do-it-yourself personnel manual construction kits. Let a person specializing in labor relations put together your manual and update it every year. (See below, pages 120-122).

Operations Operations moves your practice. It's comprised of the following segments:

Services that determine the type of scheduling you want for your practice; set up the flow of patients through your office; establish a system of good will and credibility with suppliers; install an inventory control system; arrange for you and your staff to attend seminars; and create a statistical information system to monitor your clinic's performance.

Sales and Marketing that define the market for your services; analyze your competitors; assess your patient's needs; implement patient education programs; and construct patient feedback systems measuring sources and effectivity.

Promotions that plan, budget, and execute your advertising campaign; develop press releases and other publicity programs; and initiate personal contact programs that reach out to your community.

Finances If your eyes roll back into your head when discussing finances, find an advisor you can trust. If you are not an expert on finances, turn over everything you don't understand to a CPA or tax attorney. As your financial knowledge increases, take back some of the financial planning. Spend money now on projects that will save money in the future. Contract out most of your financial work, including bookkeeping, whenever your time would be more productive doing non-financial work. Sign all the checks so you know where the money is being spent. Carefully go over the Profit & Loss statements produced by your CPA's office. To have proper control, you must keep your fingers on the financial pulse of your practice. You must know everything about the flow of your money in and out of your practice.

Finances are comprised of two areas:

General Bookkeeping. This scrutinizes financial statements to understand your cash flow.

Carefully monitor your tax obligations, especially if you pay payroll taxes. I've seen some offices shut down faster than a PBS mind watching an MTV channel when they neglected to pay their federal payroll taxes.

Financial Planning. The most important element of financial planning is your cash flow. You can be making a profit and still go under if you run out of liquid cash assets. The planning for the future use of your cash is of equal importance. Cash is the fuel that runs your practice. When it is gone, your trip is over! (Cash flow and how to chart it is covered later in this book.)

Ethics are nothing but reverence for life.
−Albert Schweitzer

3

Powerful Ethics: The Keystone Of A Strong Practice

Ethics has been defined as, "A system of moral principles." A moral principle defines the difference between the right and wrong way to perform an action. Here's where the problems arise: what's right and wrong? Philosophers have been arguing the difference between right and wrong for centuries.

Every day a doctor is faced with many decisions. Judgments have to be made concerning his or her patients, practice, and life. These decisions are not always clear. Seemingly insignificant decisions made today sometimes drastically affects life tomorrow. Ethics always seemed to be so ethereal!

Since ethics is so important in the decision-making process, a practice manager needs clear instructions to steer them in the proper direction. One excellent guide for the business owner who wants to operate under lucid, moral guidelines is the Rotary Four-Way Test.

The Four-Way Test was developed by a Rotarian during the Depression. He used it as a statement of his company's operating policy. It is now used as an ethical commitment for all Rotarians around the world. Hold all decisions up to the light of these four

> **The Rotarian Four-Way Test**
>
> Is it the truth?
> Is it fair for all concerned?
> Will it build good will and better friendships?
> Will it be beneficial to all concerned?

tests If you get four affirmative answers, chances are your decision will be ethical.

The freshness and validity of the Four-Way Test remains as powerful today as it was back in 1932. I have not seen a better set of ethical guidelines to run my practice or my life. Use these guidelines to make proper decisions that will stand up proudly to future scrutiny.

I know I made a decision, I just forgot where I put it!
　　　　　　　　　　　　　　　　　　　　　　–Proverb

4

Four Easy Steps To Decision-Making

If you want your practice to fail…Procrastinate! As the ad in the paper said, "The next meeting of the Procrastinator's Club has been postponed." Don't postpone the growth and prosperity of your practice. Decide what you want to do then do it!

There is no magic to becoming *a decisive, effective* manager. Success derives from the ability to make timely decisions and deal with whatever results occur. Chiropractors who make wild decisions without rational thought will seriously hurt their practice. Ego-based decisions will turn a practice into a top always spinning around at a frantic pace but not really going anywhere!

Most people new to management forget they have been making decisions all their lives. Getting up in the morning is a decision; driving a car is a constant series of decisions. Just going about our daily lives forces us to make numerous decisions. Most of the time we do them automatically and accurately.

Though we are not usually aware of it, we use a step-by-step process whenever we have to make a decision. As a manager, you can formalize this process into four easy steps:

Step One: Define The Full Problem. Do not jump to a conclusion when you have only a partial picture of the problem. Treat it as you would a patient. Look at all facets and, as in examining a patient, do not assume you know the full extent of a problem until you have thoroughly examined it from all sides.

Step Two: Delineate Every Plan "B" You Can Think Up! Bring your staff into the decision-making process. How many different ways can all of you devise to resolve the problem? When you and your staff are thinking up solutions, do not screen out any ideas no matter how bizarre they might seem. Do not hinder anyone's thought process by editing the initial suggestions. Get them all listed on a blackboard or flip chart. When there are no more ideas, then start editing out the obviously unworkable ideas. You'll end up with an excellent list of possible solutions.

Step Three: Prioritize Your Possible Solutions and Their Consequences. Hold your judgements until you evaluate them using a Priority List. Utilizing the Ben Franklin list (see Chapter 6), examine your solutions and see if they fit into your planning. By prioritizing, answers will "pop" right off the page. Choose the answer that best suits the defined mission and goals of your practice.

Step Four: Commit And Control! Implement your chosen solution, then monitor the resulting data. If your solution looks promising, you might have to "fine-tune" it to better fit within your goal parameters. Don't sweat the mistakes. If 51% of your decisions are good for your practice, you'll have steady progress.

That's all there is to making strong, effective decisions!

Some Tips To Help You Avoid Procrastinating

Don't set your performance bar too high for the task at hand. Raise your expectations in increments. It'll keep you from feeling besieged by the unrealistic expectation of accomplishing a particular task. For example, when I set up a car for a race, I adjusted the carburetors, suspension and tire pressures in small increments. Trying to attain a perfect setup in one big adjustment will cause major problems.

• If you have a goal of xxx patients visits per week, approach that goal in measurable increments. Spread your expectations out over a reasonable time period and set target dates for completion. When you believe your goal or objective can be accomplished, it'll be easier to make those necessary decisions.

• Be certain whatever you're trying to accomplish is a necessity. If you were roped into a task because you couldn't say no or if you are trying to do something you absolutely abhor, see if you can delegate out the portion you dislike. Then, set parameters for your future acceptance of those tasks abhorrent to you.

• Change your scenery. If you keep walking around a task without touching it, change the physical aspects of that task. Try a different time of the day to work on it. Try doing it outside rather than inside or in a group setting rather than in private. Turning on the radio works for some people and turning off for others.

• If you really, really don't like the task, have someone else do it. I maintain my front lawn at home, a service maintains the hilly side. I disliked doing a physical inventory, I had a capable staff member handle that task.

Let It Go! Did you know that according to the Small Business Administration, most small businesses do not have a formal organizational plan? Many clinic owners do many jobs that should have been delegated to their employees. They have difficulty letting go of their authority! Most small business owners feel that, "I can do the job better than anyone!" The problem is this: when you are doing your employees job, you are neglecting your own work.

A doctor once complained to me that he wasn't getting his phone messages in a timely manner. A quick investigation revealed that when his clinic phone rang, it would be picked up by the closest staffer. Messages were written on any available paper scrap, then, if the message-taker was busy, that scrap was placed on the nearest surface. No one had been delegated the responsibility to get phone messages to the doctor.

To correct this problem, responsibility for answering the phone was given to a primary and one backup employee. A message pad was used with that message placed in a "Doctor's Message Box." The problem disappeared. Not only was someone now responsible, they now knew it!

If you can learn and apply proven management techniques to run your office and take the time to train your staff, you will be an effective and successful manager. The doctor who assumes firm management of his clinic will drive it forward and upward into a future world filled with net profit and pleased patients.

What are you waiting for?

5

How To Delegate Rather Than Relegate

An effective manager is able to flow with changes in his operating environment which includes training subordinates, then delegating responsibilities to them. Be aware of the difference between relegate and delegate. When you relegate responsibility, you give up authority to your subordinate. When you delegate, your subordinate represents you while you maintain authority. Obviously, you want to delegate rather than relegate.

Let's illustrate this important difference by looking at insurance and collections.

If the employee is running the department without any supervision from the doctor, then the employee is in charge. As a result, the doctor has relegated his authority to that person. He no longer controls the insurance and collections functions. Unfortunately, I've observed this phenomenon in too many practices.

The doctor who is unfamiliar with insurance billing is reluctant to be involved. Instead of learning enough about this department to properly supervise it, the doctor stays away to perform other, more comfortable duties. The doctor is now gambling that the employee will be fully motivated to achieve the practice's goals. Not likely! The odds are better for that doctor to win the lottery.

> ### *Three Keys To Delegating*
>
> • Develop strong channels of communication between you and your team. Don't send strictly negative messages. A congratulatory pat on someone's back will have far more impact than a punch to their arm telling them they messed up.
>
> • Be truthful and encourage your employees to be truthful in return. The flow of *honest* information and suggestions should go in both directions. Otherwise, it is dictatorial, not healthy.
>
> • Be impartial. Give equal and consistent treatment to all everyone in your practice. Nothing can destroy a smooth practice than the perception of unfairness or favoritism.

Try This Example To properly manage an area of his practice, a doctor must have an overview of how that area operates and what results are expected. The easiest way is to absorb the data from that area in small increments. Each day, spend an hour observing, helping and occasionally conversing with the responsible person in that area, in this case, the insurance department. There are several benefits to this:

Your interest will be appreciated by the insurance person. *That* employee knows you are busy; therefore, when you take time to learn their department in a non-threatening and respectful manner your employee is flattered by the attention and you garner an education. Both sides win!

By absorbing the insurance information in small increments, you'll not experience information overload. You'll also be able to discuss your prior day's experience. This prevents you from going too long carrying unanswered questions.

Reducing the time it takes to perform a task is another good reason to delegate. It also creates a better bond between you and your staff as they realize you trust them to handle certain situations.

By delegating, you'll have more time to cross-train your staff members in further tasks you do not have time to perform. The cumulative results of your delegating activities will allow you to be a better manager and leave you time to focus on projects that really need your personal attention.

And, by using this method, you'll understand the responsibilities you are delegating. Knowledge of a delegated responsibility allows you to manage rather than perform thereby allowing you to personally address your higher priority tasks.

*When you have to make a choice and
don't make it, that in itself is a choice.*

–William James

6

Prioritize Before You Decide

Some managers have difficulty making decisions. We've all observed decision-makers waffle and wobble and walk around in circles trying to make a decision. Eventually, they end up not making it. That's error by omission, which is just as damaging as error by commission. If you do nothing, you will have a problem. So, at least take a chance and make a decision! Even if you're guessing, there's a 50% chance you'll be right.

The competent manager doesn't fear making mistakes and makes decisions with confidence and forethought because he has thought out the options. If a mistake is made, the manager doesn't agonize but learns and continues forward. No one enjoys making a mistake! Just don't let it mess up your future decisions! A successful manager will try to avoid repeating mistakes, but knows that, if a lesson can be learned, subsequent decisions will have a higher degree of relevance and accuracy.

If you use a system for the decision-making process, it eventually becomes ingrained and automatic. One tried and true system was allegedly used by Benjamin Franklin to look at the pros and cons of a situation before he made his decision. Let's check it out.

List Your Priorities

Competent managers consistently prioritize during their examination of any situation. You probably have unknowingly participated in this thought process.

The elements of a prioritized list must be in their real context (students of justification, rationalization and denial need not apply). When real elements are analyzed and prioritized, the decision-making process becomes less complex.

Use a priority list to make a decision on a situation or problem that has a bunch of confusing variables. When you're having trouble deciding which solution to choose, don't just flip a coin or grab the first possibility that comes to mind. That misstep will throw you down management's stairs. Instead, use "Ben's List," a technique that is attributed to Benjamin Franklin.

To construct the list, draw a vertical line down the center of sheet of paper, making two columns. Place the *pros* in one column, and the *cons* in the other (see the example on the next page). It is easier to visualize the situation you are considering and proceed to a decision when all the elements are listed.

For example, suppose your problem is: "Patients complain they are waiting too long for treatment." The answer is to reduce the patient's waiting time. Since there are several ways to resolve this problem, a *pro* and *con* list will help you decide on a solution.

The first step in constructing the list is to write down all the possible solutions:

- Expand the clinic's treatment hours.
- Augment the front desk staff.
- Bring more doctors to the practice.
- Reduce the number of scheduled patients.
- Increase the number of adjusting spaces.
- Reduce the amount of time the doctor spends with each patient.
- Devise a more efficient flow of patients through the office.
- Redesign the office layout.
- Limit new patients to special time slots.
- Have time set aside for emergencies.

Now that you have a list of possible solutions for the "patient waiting" problem, start with the first item on the your list, "Increase Treatment Hours." List all the reasons you can think of for and against this particular solution.

The strengths and weaknesses of each possible solution are listed for comparison. Base your decision about that possible solution not only by the number of pro and con items but also by the weight of the items.

Solution: Increase Treatment Hours

Arguments to Increase (PRO)	Arguments Against an Increase (CON)
There is room in the schedule to open the office an additional half to one full day	The Front Desk staff would lose the down time they use to catch up on their paperwork
There would be more available time for new patients	The extra hours would drive up labor costs
The current patient load would be spread over a longer time period thereby reducing patient waiting time	The doctor's community outreach marketing programs would be reduced due to his spending more time in the office
By adding office hours, there would be intermittent open time in the schedule for paperwork	Patients get used to certain hours and might not take advantage of the longer hours

A Ben Franklin List

For example, being able to spend more time on receivables is an added benefit, so this pro would carry more weight than the doctor's current community activities. Because each pro and con is specific to your practice, you must assign the weighting.

To obtain a clear pictures of your decision possibilities, analyze all of the proposed solutions like the partial example above. Some items will be quickly dismissed with minimal thought because, at this time, they might be unrealistic. Examples might be adding doctors or reducing patients per hour. Others will require research such as redesigning office space or changing patient processing procedures. The idea is to get all the possibilities gathered in one place so they can be examined and discussed systematically.

It is always best, after analyzing a complex situation, to let the thoughts incubate in your subconscious for a period of time. During this period, you and your staff will better arrange that data. Upon re-analysis, you'll have a stronger list from which to make your decisions.

To be an effective, successful manager, the doctor/owner must be able to recognize, then analyze, an ever-changing business environment and then to revise operating strategies so you can remain a successful entity. Prioritized problem solving is one of the powerful tools a manager can utilize to maintain a successful service entity.

*Acquire new knowledge whilst thinking over the
old, and you may become a teacher of others.*
—Confucius

7

Practice Basics Worth Repeating

Starting a practice is easier than keeping it growing. There are close to a million small business startups every year. These businesses are started by people who are looking for relevance in their lives. They want to make changes benefitting their society. They don't want to spend their lives working for someone else. So, with fire in their bellies, desire in their eyes, and knowledge in their heads, they start their business. Strengthened by all their motivations, these small businessmen (and women) have plenty of "juice" to get their dreams started. It's the long haul, however, that slowly, relentlessly chisels away at their resolve.

To keep any business going, including a chiropractic office, you can't sit back after startup and "ride the wave" of your past accomplishments. To keep your practice growing and prospering, you must possess and utilize the basic elements. You must:

- Maintain the fire and passion you had at startup. Don't let the daily details of running your practice grind you down. Constantly review your goals
- Learn to shut the doors (or get a relief doctor); go out and play. For the long haul, the right combinations of play, work, and family must be factored into your life
- Have a group of people you trust who you can bounce ideas off of and receive ideas from

• Keep up with the latest in your chiropractic community. There's an abundance of new research being produced almost daily. Being well-versed in all that is new will keep your professional outlook sparkling and vibrant.

• Develop and follow your financial planning. Reacting to financial situations is a hard and stressful way to run a practice. It is much easier to see the hills you must cross and prepare for your crossing than to stumble onto them in the dark.

• Above all, the supporting structure of your practice growth should be our familiar friends, The Basics (see below).

I attended many years of management seminars. The majority of the seminar time was spent discussing subjects like how to launch a practice, how to get your practice out of trouble, and how to use the newest gadgets being sold at that seminar. There weren't all that many meaningful discussions on how to keep a practice alive and growing after startup.

Just as we must learn how to work the pedals before we can drive safely, we need to learn how to apply the basics to our practice management in order to drive it successfully.

The Basics In order for a practice to grow, the essential foundational elements must be present upon which you then build your practice. Review these basics and use them to evaluate the strength of your practice. So, let's start!

Practice Location. This is an obvious and sometimes overlooked necessity. A nice looking office in a pleasant location is excellent and constant advertising. Whether we had single or multiple clinics, it always seemed to give that clinic an "edge" to be visible to the passing public. If your office itself cannot be positioned visibly, establish conspicuous signs leading prospective patients into your clinic.

Traffic Flow. Spend a little time observing the amount of traffic in the vicinity of your proposed clinic. If at all possible, contact your local government to obtain traffic demographics pertaining to the area of your proposed office. Also, check traffic flow in both directions as it passes your location. See if it's easy for a vehicle on the opposite side of the street to park close to the office. Visualize a patient, having trouble just walking, getting from their car to the entrance of your office.

Ground Floor. If you don't have that ground-floor location, make sure there is elevator service to your office. Can you imagine a patient with severe lumbar spasms trying to crawl up the stairs to your office? I know of colleagues who have excellent practices established in hard-to-get-to areas that are above the ground floor. But they are exceptions. Removing as many barriers as possible will always be to your advantage.

Patient Referrals. How one goes about getting those new patient referrals would fill another book and is well-documented in both practice start-up literature and seminars. We have all heard everyone's favorite way to generate referrals; however, most practice management consultants agree that internal referrals are the best and the most economical way to go about getting new patients.

Internal referrals are best generated through patient education. Patients can be educated in groups or individually. It is much more efficient to give group talks, Back schools and similar events. To educate each patient as they pass through your office is inefficient and limits your practice growth. Aside from the talks in your office, expanding them to community organizations will be indispensable in establishing your credibility and the scope of what you can accomplish as a chiropractor.

How many of your patients know the scope of your talents and what your profession can do to help them? Usually, patients have a narrow understanding of what you can provide. When you have a chance to expand their thinking, they then will refer friends with other types of health concerns.

It is beneficial to your practice when a current patient speaks highly of your talents and whatever else they admire in your practice. When a prospective patient has heard someone speaking well of your office and then calls you, they are already convinced that chiropractic has a good possibility of helping with their problem.

Name Recognition. During our early years in practice, we tried various names for our offices. The most effective was using my own name on the clinic signs. Name recognition is greatly enhanced by the use of your picture in ancillary advertising.

Your picture in the newspaper, on TV, or in the theaters adds validity to your professional presence. (This is not applicable if your picture is hanging in the post office) Even though you paid to have your picture published, it authenticates you as a legitimate entity. As you move through your community, it multiplies the effectiveness of your advertising.

Your Personal Image. The first time you see a patient, you have about ten seconds to give your new patient the impression they made the right choice in a chiropractor. The image you project to your patients and the public can hinder or enhance your success. What makes this even more difficult is that each community has different standards of perception. For example, the acceptable image in the beach area is not the same as what might be accepted in a logging camp community. You need to be accepted in your community to be successful; however, you must be honest to yourself.

Next to my family and profession, racing was an important part of my life. Yet, I did not allow my racing activities to be the defining aspect of my image because patients didn't come to my office because I won trophies. They needed someone they could trust who had the expertise to help them with their health needs. You must maintain your unique personality, at the same time, reflect an expert, ethical attitude to your public. Your professional image is based upon what you project to the public.

Your Clinic Image. Your image is composed of several components. Patient contact is just one component of the image-making process; your professionalism, the conditions in and around your office, your reputation and your style of operations all combine to portray an image to the public. Let's look at some of the essential aspects of the image picture.

With the current trend toward open adjusting areas, privacy while adjusting is becoming less of an issue. For those of you who use individual rooms, assure the privacy of your patient- doctor conversations by soundproofing adjustment room walls. This will build a comfort level during treatment.

The majority of offices I've visited appeared clean and neat, however, there were doctors who were unaware of the dirty conditions *outside* their offices. Neglected landscaping, filthy parking facilities, dirty windows, defective signage and malfunctioning entrance doors all detract from your positive image. Normally, I would enter my clinic using a private door, however, once a week I would park in my patient's area and enter my clinic using the patient's entrance. This routine gave me a patient's perspective of my "Office Look." By following this routine, you'll easily rectify neglected maintenance problems before they become cumbersome.

Be aware of your clinic's ambience. Look at the inside of your clinic as would a patient. Without intellectualizing, what is your first impression? Is it the image you want to project? Since I wanted to attract patients involved with racing, I had a wall and shelving which displayed trophies and pictures of that genre. However, I didn't want to be out of balance, so I also had a wall which displayed all my degrees, continuing education certificates, and association memberships to show my continuing efforts to stay current within my profession. Another wall displayed community awards, club presidents plaques and other indicators of my local involvements.

Be aware of the temperature inside your office by observing your staff and patients. Their comfort takes priority over your own.

Usually an office is too cold because the temperature is set to the level of comfort for the doctor and staff. Remind yourself that you're running around while your patients are not.

Take a hard look at your equipment. If you're not proud of what you see then recover, repair or replace. Old equipment will continue to project a professional image if they're kept clean, updated and recovered when wear turns to tattered.

While you're looking over your equipment, look at your staff then yourself. Does everyone look like they belong working in a doctor's office? I allowed staff to pick out their preferences in jackets from a catalog which I provided (This keeps the cost within your specified parameters).

You should be able to tell the players without a score card, and that goes for the doctor as well.

How much harder does the doctor have to work to project his professionalism when he greets patients wearing cute summer shorts or gaudy, excessive, or super-expensive jewelry? Since I don't like wearing ties, I wore a colored jacket and comfortable slacks in my clinic. The only time I deviated from being suitably dressed was during off-hour emergency visits. Whatever style clothing you wear, just be aware of what it portrays. What images are you projecting to your patients?

Office operations are discussed later in this book; however, be aware that the way you or staff answers phones or talks during office hours add to your patient's perception of your image. What image does a gum-cracking, sloppily-dressed, patient-ignoring receptionist show to your patients versus a warm-greeting, neat-appearing person?

The cost of creating an image is simply awareness; the cost of presenting a poor image is simply immense!

How you are perceived by your public is as important as being recognized! This is especially true during your first years in practice. After you are established, you are less likely to be damaged by minor personal idiosyncracies.

The other chiropractors in town worked very hard at establishing their names as professionals and good citizens. This approach succeeds! As an example, when we first established our practice in town, the local newspaper would never use the title "Doctor" when mentioning any chiropractor. By the time I retired, the newspaper had begun to use that proper and respectful title. Thanks to the consistent community work practiced by these chiropractors to establish *their* professional chiropractic image, recognition slowly surfaced in the eyes of the public and te media.

In free countries, every man is entitled to express his opinions and every other man is entitled not to listen.

–G. Norman Collie

8

Free Advice: Worth What You Pay For It

When you examine your managerial strengths and weaknesses, you may discover deficiencies in areas such as financial planning *or* accounting. After examining possible solutions, you may eventually chose to use outside contractors to help you out.

You may encounter failures and disasters with some of your consultant choices. If you find your outside consultant is not performing to your needs, then do not hesitate to shop for another. I found the best consultants were found through referrals from respected professionals in other fields.

One concept is particularly important to remember. If you find an advisor in accounting, advertising, practice management, or office layout who has the ability to competently guide you in successful operations, their fees are secondary to their contribution to your success. Conversely, if you choose an advisor who is incapable of contributing toward the advancement of your success, terminate the relationship and don't waste any more money!

Somewhere around five years into my practice, after I had armed myself with the basics, I was able to dispense with most of my paid advisors. One consultant I continue using to this day is a tax attorney. Although he is important in helping me put together a clear picture of my business operations, I still make all final decisions.

Remember, no matter how erudite your advisor appears to be, his opinions are just that. His opinions! The picture he sees will be colored by his life-experiences. The actions he advises you to take will affect your life-experience, not his. Therefore, analyze your advisors' information and recommendations but make your own decisions regarding your next course of action! With practice and time, your final decisions will be more relevant. After all, who better knows how to race the course than the driver?

9

Why You Need A Mission Statement

After several years in practice, you should have already asked yourself, "What is my mission?" Why am I here? If your answer is "to make a lot of money," or "to be my own boss," or "to avoid being an associate," you are not expressing a manageable mission. You are expressing a denigrating desire.

A good mission statement tells why your business exists and defines its market niche.

Therefore, the first two questions to ask yourself are:

- Why did I open my practice?
- Where will I implement the services of my practice?

The answers to these questions will start you on the road to constructing your mission statement.

Now, ask yourself these questions:

- What do you want your clinic to accomplish?
- What impact do you want your practice to make in your community?
- How much of yourself are you willing to invest toward the achievement of your mission?

The answers to these and other questions will help formulate your mission. Once it is constructed, you will then have a foundation from which your business will build, grow, and prosper.

Lofty, wordy mission statements are very difficult to relate or convey to your patients and staff. Working with a complex mission statement multiplies the work you have to go through to accomplish your goals. An over-complicated, complex mission statement is one reason why only five percent of our population ever set goals.

How do you explain your mission during a staff meeting if that mission statement is enigmatic, complicated, and difficult to understand? If you hear your staff or patients tell you, "Gee, that sounds wonderful. What does it mean?" consider coming down from Mount Olympus to simplify your mission statement.

It is important for your staff and patients to easily understand your purpose, It is equally important for you to get them involved and in agreement with your purpose. They will then help and encourage you to set the goals necessary for its accomplishment.

Your mission statement should be simple and realistic. It delineates the reason for your professional existence and outlines the area which you want to affect. Your mission statement will guide you into the conception, preparation, and targeting of your goals.

One example of a simple, realistic mission statement is: "To positively affect the health of my community."

Remember, it must be easy for you and your staff to visualize. It must be realistic, honest, and true to you, not some "political" statement that you think will sound good to the public.

If your original declaration is too lofty to be practical, you must re-construct it within the parameters of your capability. Shooting for the moon is not unrealistic, just construct some stairs in between to help you get there.

If your clinic is experiencing difficulties reaching its goals and objectives, perhaps it's time to re-evaluate and modify your mission. Your mission, like your goals (which we will discuss later), could be a "grand idea." You and your staff must, however, believe it is possible to achieve. If, later, you find the moon too close, modify your mission and shoot for Mars!

Your mission is a fundamental aspect of your purpose as a chiropractor!

A Side Benefit

Your mission statement is also an excellent tool to give your financial institution a clearer picture of the direction you intend to take your practice. Establishing a respected banking relationship is a valuable card to hold for the future. Communicating with your financial partners will be enhanced if you can show them an articulate financial plan for the future of your practice.

During one of our financial learning periods, we made a catastrophic error which placed a lot of pressure on our cash reserves. (Yep, wiped them out!) I assembled all my "stuff" (Mission statement, goals, objectives statistics, and other pertinent information) and visited my local bank. I showed the loan officer our vision for the future of our practice. That information, coupled with graphs of our clinic's operations, greatly helped to communicate the financial needs of my practice.

All my "Show & Tell" established, in the mind of that bank officer, that we were working toward being a productive member in our community.

When those in your sphere of influence begin to understand and agree to what you plan to accomplish, they will willingly join in helping your team. Their help will smooth your road to the winner's circle!

*Aim at the sun, and you may not reach it;
but your arrow will fly far higher than if
aimed at an object on a level with yourself.*

–Joel Hawes

10

How To Set Goals

Goals? We Don't Need No Stinking Goals! (Apologies to *The Treasure Of Sierra Madre*.)

When you started your practice, you dreamt of the mountain top your practice was going to reach. Did you just dream it, or did you set goals to accomplish that dream? Is your practice achieving the heights you wanted to reach, or are you still stuck working in the valley?

To be a winner, you must set goals. A goal is a general statement of accomplishment. One example of a goal would be "to increase my intake of new patients." Another example would be "to strengthen my cash reserves." A third example would be "to increase the number of patient visits." From these general areas, you will develop specific objectives.

An objective is the bulls-eye you and your staff want to hit! If you are going to hit that bulls-eye, you must know how to specifically state the objective so that it is realistic and achievable. You have to know where you are starting so that you can measure your progress. Finally, you must have a time line so that you know when it is achieved.

If one of your goals is "an increase in our new patients," then one of your objectives should be, "A ten percent increase in new patients during the next ninety days."

When you set your sights on an objective, drive toward it with all the power you possess until it is achieved. Don't deviate from your course!

It surprised me to discover how many doctors told me they operated without goals or objectives. Some doctors felt they were not a necessary element to a successful practice. Some doctors started working with goals and objectives, but, for whatever reasons, soon lost focus and drive. Those doctors felt constant goal focus was not as important as hard work. I strongly disagree.

How do you know the direction you must travel if you don't have a goal? How do you know if you've made any progress in a direction unless you have a goal to accomplish?

Properly set goals will lead you to develop specific objectives. Both must be kept firmly in focus. Don't lose sight of either until they are reached, modified, or discarded. If your practice doesn't seem to be progressing, check your goals and objectives. If you can't "see" them, you'll not accomplish them!

Ask yourself, have you:

• Made plans which will guide your practice through the coming years?
• Formalized goals and objectives that will direct your practice to better serve your community?
• Written down your objectives to give you targets for personal and clinic accomplishments?

All competitive events have goals and objectives. Whether you like it or not, when you opened your practice, you entered into a competition. Not with your colleagues or other health professional, but with yourself! Many chiropractors get whiplash trying to see what other offices are doing. That shouldn't be your focus. It'll distract and delay the progress of your practice. You should set your own standards and be your strongest competitor!

The other day, a fellow chiropractor and I were discussing methods for visualizing goals. We agreed that writing down objectives derived from goals enhances the visualization process. The doctor said he wrote all of his goal objectives on small pieces of paper. He'd post those papers inside his car and around his office. This chiropractor finds it effective to even stick them on the mirrors in his home and under his pillow. All of his goals and objectives have been accomplished or exceeded. He's constantly setting new levels of accomplishments for himself and his clinic. Try it! This concept works!

A goal remains a wish until you take action toward its accomplishment. Taking action will prompt the setting of the objectives to accomplish those goals. Many of your colleagues have probably told you what they wanted their practices to accomplish. Yet, when you asked what action plans they had for achieving those desires, you got "The check's in the mail" look. Unless you get off your Southern end and move in a Northerly direction, those "someday goals" are merely dreams and wishes.

How To Set Goals And Objectives?

Goals are generic. They are not action statements. They are achievements. Their function is to lead you to the stepping stones to your goals, your objectives. Objectives should contain several important elements to be effective.

State them in a specific manner. Let's examine specificity as it applies to travel instructions. Suppose you stop on a country road, ask a local for directions, and hear something like, "Well Ol' buddy, you go down a-ways to the first, uh, maybe second barn then turn kinda left toward some field that was just plowed" and so on. How helpful would you find directions like these?

Your mind, including your subconscious, works best with detailed information, much like a computer. Similar metaphors apply, especially "garbage in-garbage out"! Write your objectives with enough detail to clearly indicate the road you want to travel.

Make them tangible. You must be able to "see" it. Otherwise, it will be like trying to find your destination on a blank road map. I have trouble visualizing numbers. When I have to understand sets of numbers, I write them down. If you only vaguely "see" your goals, they are not "real." Your mind will have trouble grasping the concepts they represent. So, make sure your goals are tangible and have a solid image in your mind.

Make them attainable, but a challenge. To gain benefit from any *physical* exercise, you have to challenge your muscles. If you make the exercise too easy, you gain no benefit. The same applies to your "business muscles." It would be a waste of time to set a goal that states, "I'm going to wake up tomorrow morning." There's no challenge therefore no progress will occur.

Don't make your goals too easy to accomplish. To advance yourself, you must push your personal limits. I relate the concept of limits to seeing how fast a race car could get through a turn. I'm always looking for the "edge" or limits of adhesion. When testing my car out on the track before a race, I "push the corner" until the car starts to slide out of control. I'm constantly surprised to see how much deeper my car will go through a turn when my comfort zone is pushed to its limit.

Your direction, just like an unused muscle, will atrophy unless you move past your present limits and into new territory. Making your practice advance means moving it forward. It takes more "mind muscle" to move your practice onto its next level than you might currently possess. The only way to make that muscle grow is to challenge it just like a weight lifter gets larger and stronger by steadily increasing his weights.

If you want to grow, you must set goals that will be a challenge.

Make them measure to your objective. You must have a system that informs you where you started and how far you have gotten. Let's say you're driving to a location that's 300 miles down the road. You've got two days to get there, therefore, you can drive 150 miles a day, sight-see along the way, and still get to your objective on time.

But, what if you don't have a speedometer or odometer and are driving on side roads with no mileage markers? Where are you at any given time of your driving day? You probably won't have a clue. You need to have measurements indicating the progress toward your objectives. Statistics, charts, or mini-objectives are just several examples of methods to measure your progress. However you set up the measuring systems, they are essential to show you progress or the lack of it. Don't be discouraged by lack of progress. It is also good. When you are aware of no progress, you'll change the way you're doing things. Your measurements will then be able to show you the success of those changes.

Make a definite time to reach your objective. Without a definite time-line to reach your objective, the urgency for attainment disappears. The chances for accomplishing your objective also greatly diminishes.

Based upon your objectives, you and your staff can devise and implement a plan or strategy that outlines the actions you'll take to accomplish your objectives and sets firm deadlines for their accomplishment. Achieve your objectives and you will attain your goals. When attained, just reset for your next level of accomplishment.

Goals followed by objectives are the basic tools preventing your dreams and desires from decaying into nightmares and yearnings. Without them and action plans for their actualization, you'll be too busy keeping up with yesterday to plan for tomorrow.

Mark Twain said, "Even if you're on the right track, you'll get run over unless you keep moving." Goals will get you on the right track. You have to keep moving toward your objectives; otherwise, you're going to get run over by the next train.

The very fact that you are setting goals starts the magic! Remember, your goals should be used to guide your personal as well as your business life. Otherwise, your life becomes unbalanced, and an unstable personal life will seriously affect your business operations. Your goals will help guide you toward the attainment of your wishes and desires. If your wishes and desires are cast within a framework of morality, ethics, and compassion, you will be a noble winner.

*Plan and work are synergistic,
stronger together than apart.*
—Engineering Proverb

Blueprint For Success: Your Business Plan

Plan is not a four-letter word

Never, under any circumstances, take a sleeping pill and a laxative on the same night.
—Dave Barry

Most chiropractors are excellent technicians. They have learned about and know how to apply the tecnhical aspects of the profession. They know about the sleeping pills and laxatives and they know what happens when they take them. But far too many of them still take them anyway. They "mess up" by not planning for the regular growth of their businesses.

In 1995, *Entrepreneur* magazine conducted a survey of businesses that failed within the first five years. One of the most important reasons was "the inability of management to properly plan, reach decisions, and act upon them." This is a particular danger for chiropractors, most of whom prefer to be hands-on players and not desk jockeys.

A second cause of failure is unanticipated success. Chiropractors who grow too fast can find that their resources have been over-extended and blow the doors shut on a promising practice faster than the wind from the houses of Congress.

Either way, more chiropractors need to become proficient in the planning and management of their practices. No one is more qualified to lead their practices to success, and part of leading is knowing the big picture. Consider your role as the driver of a car. If you were only a carburetor technician, you'd only need to master the technical aspects of adjusting the mixture of air and fuel. But as the owner of your car, you also need to know how and where to drive it. That takes planning and forethought.

Like driving to Aunt Millie's house for Thanksgiving or Malibu for the summer, becoming a successful chiropractor (or lawyer or publisher, for that matter) involves more than turning the engine over, putting the seat belt on, and hitting the road. It involves asking a number of questions and determining the actions you will take for each answer.

As a chiropractor you might ask questions like:

• What areas of my practice do I need to strengthen?
• What strategic plans will I need to make to compete in the changing marketplace?
• What additional education do I need to enhance the growth of my practice?

The answers you get will help you "drive" your practice over and around the obstacles you and the outside world throw in your path. You may not be able to control external events like changes in the economy or seasonal distractions, but you still need to plan for them, just as you need to plan for gasoline, food, and pit stops on your drive. Once you determine your destination and figure out how you will get there, then you can get off your duff and start driving with more confidence that you will get there.

Five Easy Questions One of the primary ingredients in the success formula is planning. Not sitting at your desk biting your nails and worrying, but real planning! You need to have a business plan. As a small business owner, you might feel intimidated when asked to write a business plan. Don't be discouraged! It is easy as long as you understand it's purpose and it's guidelines.

The Business Plan is your plan to be used for your own purpose. There is no right or wrong way to write it. However, do not let anyone else write it for you. In the course of answering the five questions listed below, you will be putting together a business plan. You will be examining both the strengths and weaknesses of your practice. You will provide priorities and the direction toward accomplishment of your mission and its goals. By the time you finish writing down your business plan, you'll better understand who you are and what you must do to achieve your dreams.

A business plan can also be used to secure outside operating capital. When I started my practice, I believed my financing should be with personal rather than borrowed funds. The reasons? Accountability and liability. I had no one to question my expenditures but myself, and I had no payment obligations to meet each month. I knew the money was hard-gained, so I wanted control over spending it.

My business plan was not written to secure outside capital. I knew if I constructed a business plan, following the standard procedure outlined below, I would be forced to examine all the basic aspects of my proposed business. Since the examination would highlight my weak areas, I wanted to face any deficiencies early and fix them. I wanted to do this before I started practice. It is best to face your plan's deficiencies early and fix them before your trip over those rocks down the road. If you are surprised later, lack of planning might turnabout and fix you!

I sincerely hope you started your clinic with a business plan in hand. If not, now is the time to put one together! True, many clinics have started without one; however, most of the thousands of successful clinics did start with a plan.

In order to formulate the plans that will include your goals for a successful clinic, you have to honestly look to yourself for some of the necessary answers. Below are the five questions you must ask yourself. The answers you derive from those questions will be your business plan.

How can I best describe my business? It is not enough to say you provide chiropractic services. A description of chiropractic and how it will benefit a patient is proper. This is not the forum, however, for an intense philosophical discussion. Make it succinct.

This is more than just saying "I provide chiropractic." Your descriptions should be written as if you were painting a word picture for someone who has never seen a chiropractic practice. Put yourself into your prospective patient's shoes. They would ask you, "What exactly is chiropractic service and what will you do to me?"

You should also describe the type of business you have; a partnership, sole proprietorship, or corporation. Is it brand new or have you taken over another's practice? Where is your office located? Is it easily accessible to the patient who is in pain and struggling to walk? Can a patient park reasonably close to the office? Can a patient visit your office during evening hours and feel safe walking from the car to the entrance of your office? How much space do you have, and is it capable of expansion? Is the area in which your office is located stable, or is it undergoing changes? Will those changes affect the demographics of your patient base?

What type of service will I be providing? Your description should cover how you intend to provide your services and how you will make sure they are more beneficial to your patients than similar services in your community. (Special techniques, reasonable fee schedules, etc.). What are your operating hours and how are they designed to best suit your prospective patients?

Who are my competitors? Whether you want to admit it, you are vying for a piece of a finite pie. Others in chiropractic and allied professions also want a piece of that pie. Whether it is a formula car race or a chiropractic office, you must know the perceived strengths and weaknesses of your opponents. No name-calling or mud-slinging! Your description should be insightful, respectful, and professional.

What is my management structure? This involves more than giving yourself a title. Giving yourself or others in your group an unnecessary title such as, "Assistant Vice-President of World Chiropractic Marketing" will not serve your purpose. The idea here is to determine who in your organization hold management responsibilities. As you now know, managing a practice requires more than your technical expertise. A successful practice will reflect smart resource management. Those resources are your staff. If you let them feel it's OK to suggest practice improvements, your practice will greatly benefit from mining that resource. Their excellent suggestions will often point you to a higher level of practice performance.

A successful chiropractic practice also reflects the ability of the doctor/owner to know his or her strengths and weaknesses. When some organizational details drove me bonkers, I hired a detail-oriented person to handle those tasks. It made my office life much more bearable and productive allowing me to concentrate on my strength, people management.

What Is My Marketing Plan? Marketing is a crucial component to the success of your practice. Simply stating that you intend to advertise or do internal marketing is insufficient. Describe the financial and organizational structure of the advertising programs you intend to put into action. For example, how much you plan to budget for advertising? In what media will you be placing your advertising?

Describe your marketing area plus any applicable demographics, keeping in mind that another key element to your marketing success is understanding your patient base. A major goal of your practice will be to fulfill the needs of your patients. To accomplish this, you should be aware of their general income level, the type of chiropractic service they will expect, and what type of services they will not tolerate.

For young offices, a three mile radius surrounding your office is a reasonable marketing area. As your practice matures, you will notice your marketing area increases, but that comes with time.

Marketing the North American continent is a great goal, but an unrealistic one, for a one-office marketing plan.

Delman Chiropractic Marketing Guide To help guide the preparation of your marketing plan, here's a guide I've used to help steer my marketing considerations.

A. Patient base—Who are they?
1. We will market to the following groups (Indicate percentage of each)
    a. General public
    b. Business
    c. Government
    d. Personal injury
    e. Worker's Comp
    f. Others

B. Competing services
1. Name(s)
    a. Years in practice
    b. Market percentage
    c. Types of Services (MD,DC,PT,etc.)
    d. Cost of service
2. Ratio of providers/population
3. How do you measure up vs competing services?
    a. List all your strengths (location, reputation, special skills, personnel, your resources)
    b. List all your weaknesses

C. Market Stability
1. Population
2. Industrial
3. Economic
4. Tax base changes
5. Personnel availability

D. Public Perception (What image do we want people to see?)
1. Expensive
2. Reasonable
3. Convenient
4. Ridiculously inexpensive
5. Has every gadget known to man
6. Tells good jokes

E. What services will we highlight?
1. Special training and skills
2. DC to the (Insert stars, football team, race car team)
3. Modern clinic

4. Speedy Hi-Lo tables
   5. Teaches lowly students

F. Fee Structure
   1. We will adopt the following fee guidelines
   2. Is our public perception in line with our fee structure?
   3. How does our fee structure align with similar competing services?
   4. Does our fee structure result in net profit?

G. Advertising/Promotion
   1. Total marketing budget
   2. Budget Allocations (percentage of each)
      a. Newspaper
      b. Yellow pages
      c. Radio
      d. Billboard
      e. Direct mail
      f. Personal contacts
      g. Slick, promotional salespeople
      h. Television

This marketing guide is user-friendly. You can delete any segments that are inapplicable to your situation and add any that will better guide your thoughts. The guide's main purpose is to help you focus the thrust of your marketing actions.

12

Duties Of A Practice Manager

A common misconception is to be a successful manager, you must be born with genetic qualities endowing you with basic management skills. Doctor, you may have the "right stuff." However, there is an educational process everyone must experience before becoming competent as a manager. When someone says, "You're a born manager," they're referring to the positive traits you show for management tasks. Possessing the requisite personality qualities allows you to learn management easier. However, managers are still trained, not born!

Below are the areas a manager must learn to proficiently control.

He or she must:

- Be capable of developing a master plan for the operation of his practice
- Determine the mission statement, goals, and objectives that are necessary for the successful growth of his practice
- Have the skills necessary to recognize when objectives are reached and be adept at re-establishing new ones
- Formulate the strategies for obtaining the goals and objectives of his practice
- Be capable of organizing the activities of his staff toward achieving his practice objectives

- Analyze, then arrive at decisive conclusions regarding, the data derived from his operations
- Be able to effectively see into the future (A good crystal ball helps).

Below are three critical areas of your practice requiring close management:

Planning, then directing, the operation of your business. You know your business and are aware of what you want to accomplish. It is not enough, however, just to plan your business, expecting it to operate without your personal direction, even if you have a competent office staff. As sure as the sun will rise tomorrow, sans proper supervision, your staff will wander off the road to your goals and objectives. You mustn't remain nailed to your desk playing executive, especially during the operating hours of your office. You have to be aware of every operating detail in your practice. This includes following up on assigned staff responsibilities. I call this Mobile Management. Here's how it works.

During patient hours and at other times when staff worked in my office, I would make it a point to "do rounds." I walked through every part of the office, checking areas for cleanliness, machine maintenance and supplies. I also observed staff interaction with patients, how they handled scheduling and so on. This was done in an obvious, not sneaky, fashion. I wanted to be seen walking around the office. I wanted staff to know I consistently checked on procedures and protocols.

If I didn't totally understand a working area of my office, I would spend extra time there until I felt comfortable with it's functions.

The majority of my desk time was during off-hours. Until you are of sufficient size to warrant hiring an office manager who can utilize "Mobile Management," your place is out in your office, not behind your desk. Even when I had an office manager, I made "rounds," just not as often.

Cash-flow. Cash-flow simply is the monies coming and going in your business. It is essential to know your future cash requirements as well as current cash expenditures. (See below.)

Most successful companies use some form of cash-flow projection. Only the extraordinary manager can carry the information in his or her head. A cash-flow budget and projection can be a complex exercise, listing every possible anticipated and actual income / expense item in your business. But gathering the cash flow data can be as simple as looking back to your prior basic income and expense items, and setting them down on paper, all to anticipate similar numbers in the future. After you reach the future time period, you write the actual numbers in a column next to your budget. You then analyze and adjust your budget for any differences. The answers will give you the details regarding the life's blood of your practice, your cash-flow.

I used an informal system which included charting all income and expenses over the years. That cyclical information allowed me to plan for low cash periods. I also kept a separate cash reserve for unforeseen expenditures, such as emergency equipment repair. If additional funds were needed, they were obtained via short-term bank loans at negotiated interest rates. The business axiom, "The best time to borrow money is when you don't need it" holds true. It is to your advantage to predict low cash periods but to borrow when you're in a strong cash position. Some of my colleagues use their credit cards in lieu of bank loans. This is not a smart business practice. Credit card financing is very expensive and should be utilized only if that loan can be paid off within thirty days or less, thus avoiding their high interest charges.

Inventory Management. How much money do you want to tie up in vitamins, appliances, literature and equipment? You'll be shocked to find how much capital you have sitting on your shelves. (We'll discuss inventory in greater detail later.)

13

Developing Yourself As A Manager

Pushing Your Limits

Man's mind, once stretched by a new idea, never regains its original dimensions.
—Oliver Wendell Holmes

How do you know how good you really are until you push yourself to your *perceived* limits? Driving your efforts past the limits of your comfort zone creates positive changes and constructive accomplishments.

In metallurgical engineering, there are two types of mechanical changes elastic and plastic. Elastic changes take place when you stretch a material no further than it is used to going (within its comfort zone). When released, that material will return to its original shape. Plastic changes take place when a material is stretched past it's comfort zone and, when released, will not return all the way back to it's original shape. Permanent change has taken place!

A competitive person, whether race driver or manager, will consistently try to improve themselves by stretching their performance levels past the edges of their comfort zone. Here again, racing parallels life's endeavors. During test sessions at a race track, I will push my car as hard as possible to check its setup. During testing, I will try raising my shift points to see if I can get a few more rpms out of my motor or hold off braking just a little longer into a turn. In other words, I look for improvement by stretching the limits of my comfort zone.

The size of your personal achievement zone is a similar situation. You can either stay huddled underneath a blanket of comfort and be elastic, always returning back to your same state (How limiting and boring!) Or, you can go past your perceived limits, expanding your world and never return to your prior state of mind.

Expanding your horizons involves changing your perception of the world. Before you can change your world, you must change yourself! Exploring the outer limits of your perceived world will give you access to an unlimited universe of greater opportunities.

Taking Risks

Running a chiropractic practice is a lot like driving a race car. Your success involves your willingness to take calculated risks.

You say that taking risks make you uncomfortable? Of course it does. Most people are unwilling to take calculated risks because they are reluctant to push the perceived comfort limits of their operating envelope. Yet for most people, the comfort zone is limited only by the same perceptions that limit their world. If you're willing to push the walls of your comfort zone, open your own practice, change your operating protocols, or present your chiropractic beliefs to an audience, you'll expand your world and more easily accomplish your goals.

Not just any risk. The best risk to take is a *calculated* risk. If your data show that you have a good chance of success, you can expect the risk to pay off. Courage may be nice to have, but courage without wisdom is foolishness. Unless courage is partnered with forethought and analysis, it invites you to deny the risk.

Denying risk reminds me of the person who jumps off a ten-story building. As he whizzes past the sixth floor, someone looks out the window and hollers, "How's it going?" The falling person yells back, "So far, so good!" Now, that is denial.

Anyone who stretches perceived boundaries and takes a calculated risk will always be ahead of someone who is afraid to take any risk at all. Don't let the fear of failure hinder your decision-making. You must be unafraid of failure if you want to take full advantage of your courage Winners are wary but they are not afraid to lose. Losers are stopped, not by failure, but by their *imagined* consequences of failure.

A character in a novel once said, "Failure is the condiment that gives success its flavor." Success does not have to be dramatic. It can be celebrated in inches. When you decide to act, you will make progress even if your decision moves you only a little closer to success.

D.A.R.E. to Risk

D.A.R.E. is an acronym to remind you of four steps that will help you take calculated risks.

- **Determine** the extent of your risk.

How far do you want to extend your personal and financial resources to make your decision work? Is the prospective gain worth the time and money it will cost?

Be aware of your chances for success and failure. When I was racing into a turn, I knew the spot on the track where I had to back off or spin out. Know how far you can go before your chances of success drastically diminish.

When you are making your decision "Ben Franklin" list, putting down everything you can think of will help you determine your chances for success or failure. Leave out as much emotion as you can. Facts work much well than fantasy.

- **Assess** your cost for taking this particular risk.

Can you afford to lose what you are going to gamble? Is second place better than not finishing the race? How much of your life do you want to tie up to make this decision work?

Will your commitment to this risk take time away from other, more productive activities?

How much money can you afford to lose without hindering the progress or growth of your practice? As the risks increase, so do the chances for failure. Set aside money for risky projects

Minimize the financial impact of a possible failure by being able to afford to lose your investment.

- **Review** your strategies before taking any risk.

Know what you are going to do before you challenge a situation. This is where your business and marketing plans come into play. When you create them, you'll ask yourself important questions. The answers to those questions will form the strategies and goals you'll use to guide your venture.

- **Eliminate** negative advice from your planning.

Do your own research, and leave the nay-saying to someone else.Chiropractic was my third career. When I decided to return to college and study Chiropractic, well-meaning relatives told me I was crazy for giving up my solid career for future uncertainties. However, before I chose my new career, I had researched the chiropractic market and talked to practitioners, so I knew the possibilities for success were excellent. My advisors meant well, but I was aware of the risks and knew that the career was well worth pursuing.

It's now time to translate all of the above to your next risky challenge. Drive through the steps. Don't stand by while the world zips past your practice! Take action to move forward. If the numbers and the facts look good to you…if you think your chances for success are good…step on the professional accelerator and make it happen!

Keeping Your Goals In Sight

You cannot depend on your eyes when your imagination is out of focus.
—Mark Twain

"Don't lose your focus!" That phrase was hammered at us at racing school until I became sick of hearing it!

But it's true. Every time I had a non-mechanical driving problem out on the track, it was because I lost my focus. The results of those lapses were sometimes very expensive. It didn't take too many of those lessons for me to get the message.

When I was chasing a car, my focus was on passing that car. All else was secondary. Only if and when that goal was accomplished was it reset. The same applies to running your clinic. After you set your goals, attack them one at a time, with total concentration and effort. Do not try and go after multiple goals at the same time. It does not work! Did you ever try to hit a nail with a hammer and, at the same time, turn your head to talk to someone? Do not dilute your approach toward attaining your goals. The results will be weak and wasted.

Thomas Edison is one of my icons and an excellent role model for goal accomplishment. He is noted for saying, "Genius is ninety-nine percent perspiration and one percent inspiration." He had a genius for focusing on a problem and not letting go until it was resolved.

While visiting the Fairfield Village / Ford Museum in Dearborn Michigan, I spent considerable time going through the replica of Edison's New Jersey laboratory. There was an impressive amount of material explaining the many methods Edison used in his various experiments. I was surprised to discover that he was known as a technologist rather than a scientist. He actually contributed very little to original scientific knowledge. Edison's goal was to reap great profits from the applications of his inventions.

The thousands of patents registered by Thomas Edison illustrate his talents in numerous areas, including business. He was an vigorous, hard-driving manager. He consistently had several teams of technicians, each concentrating its efforts on a specific problem. When that problem was resolved, they were assigned another. He knew that by setting up focus groups to work on specific problems, his results would be more dramatic than if he diluted the work of his teams on a multitude of research problems. The investigative directions of each group was personally directed by Edison. He assembled their finished work and immediately patented the completed product.

Thomas Edison was also an accomplished salesman. His forte, making presentations to financiers, resulted in substantial funding for his research groups. He admitted many of the ideas he worked on were not his. However, he felt that the originators of those ideas had given up too soon due to lack of focus and determination. He failed well over 1,000 times, testing various materials, before he finally perfected a workable filament for the incandescent light.

Edison had the ability to keep his goals and objectives firmly fixed until they were attained. He had mastered the art of totally focusing on the work at hand.

Here's a show-and-tell you can do to illustrate that point. Take the flat of your hand and press it on a piece of wood. Your hand does not penetrate the wood! Now, take a pin and press that on the piece of wood. It will start to penetrate into the wood! Why? The pressure of the pin was focused down to one point rather than spread out over your entire hand.

The doctors who accomplish their goals have learned to focus on them until they are achieved.

A Complacency Check

After your office has been operating a few years, you will have developed your procedures into easier, more comfortable routines. Be careful, that you haven't succumbed to the siren call of the Practice Plateau. It is a stage in your career where the panic situations have been resolved, your practice feels comfortable, and you are surviving. But, are you growing, both personally and in your practice?

Do you talk on the phone longer, letting your patients wait more than usual for your services? Have you stopped arriving at the office at least thirty minutes early to make certain it is ready to serve your patients? Are you no longer available for those emergency calls from your patients?

If this is happening, you are in the *rutzone!*

The rutzone is a synonym for a non-changing, excessively cozy, exceedingly sheltered, non-routine-changing, mind-numbing grave-with-no-ends, work-trench.

When you find yourself in the rutzone, it is time to re-evaluate the standards that guide your operations. They have become barriers to your growth rather than guidelines to your goals.

Before you rush off to frantically revise your procedures (and possibly do more harm than good), re-examine your procedures. Use the following guidelines to ensure each procedure:

• Makes sense to you
• Fits in with your mission and goals
• Works to your advantage and to the continuing betterment of yourself as well as your practice
• Allows you to modify it as you grow

- Can be changed if it is not performing within your practice guidelines.

Changing Procedures In Small Increments

In all affairs it's a healthy thing now and then to hang a question mark on the things you have long taken for granted.
—Bertrand Russell

The key to the success of any operation is in the details. The changes you'll be making will be small, incremental changes. By doing this, you'll keep from destroying whatever successful procedures you currently use. Joe Gibbs, the successful football coach and now successful race team owner uses this method. When he first evaluates a situation, he'll observe for a long time, making no changes. Then, he'll make small changes in procedures, personnel, and equipment. After just a few years owning race teams, his success is approaching that of his football career.

When we were five or six years into our practice, we noticed our "Kept Appointments" graph was in a decline. So, I spent time out at the front desk observing. The person in charge was doing a great job. No answers at that station. I didn't have any clues regarding the reason for the appointment decline until a staff member mentioned that patients seem to be waiting longer than normal. Several patients even had re-scheduled their appointments because they weren't seen close to the time of their appointment. Some patients walked out to take care of other business and didn't re-schedule.

When the decline in kept appointments was discussed at our staff meeting, everyone turned to point at me. I received the message with great clarity. The culprit was me! Between seeing patients, I was spending too much time on the phone. This may have been acceptable when I was seeing fewer patients; however, I failed to reduce my time on the phone as my practice increased.

I had been practicing in the rutzone and didn't know it! Business and nature are never in stasis. Either there is growth or decline. Since I was performing the same procedures without change or growth, that aspect of my practice was shrinking.

I curtailed my phone activities between patient visits and the curve reversed, returning to a growth track. Thank goodness for the honesty and awareness of our staff!

Methods That Will Advance Your Practice

All that is human must retrograde if it does not advance.
—Edward Gibbon

As the doctor who owns the clinic, you are the big dog on the porch. You are top management! The buck is supposed to come to a screeching halt at your desk. You're the person who must come up with creative, inspirational, and feasible solutions to practice problems.

It is natural, after several years in practice, to get "comfortable." This is dangerous, because it can stall then retrogress the growth of your practice. *When your practice growth starts to slow down*, a decision must be made. As the owner/manager, you have to make a conscious effort to raise the level of your practice. So, how do you do that? There are several routines you can institute to get you there.

Constantly question and re-evaluate your practice in all its aspects.

Be aware of what's going on in your office. This doesn't have to be a formal affair. Just keep a small portion of your awareness consistently focused on clinic operations during your normal day (If there is such a thing as a normal day). As you move around the office, if something gets your attention, don't ignore it. Your subconscious is ringing your alarm bell; listen to it and investigate.

My staff was aware I knew what was going on in the office. This kept them alert and involved. The more involved they were in office operations, the better their performance.

Periodically step into your staff's shoes. You may be surprised how well they are doing despite all their interruptions, including you.

Do this also with your patients and any one else with whom you deal in your office. Experience what it is like to be in an exam room for 15 minutes in a flimsy gown, listening to the staff laughing and having a grand time outside the door while you tap your bare foot wondering when you'll be seen by the doctor and wondering what might be wrong with you. This knowledge will greatly enhance your sensitivity to the needs of both staff and patients.

Encourage your staff to take notes. Look at both sides of your operating coin. Have them note both good and not-so-good patient relations. They should bring these notes to the weekly meetings so you can work at repeating the good things and correcting the not-so-good.

Always know the current operating status of your practice. Plan is NOT a nasty four letter word! How can you operate your clinic without a plan? How can you plan if you have no data? As a successful doctor, you already systematically gather the operating statistics of your practice such as services, collections, new patients and patient visits. I strongly recommend this be done on a weekly basis. Instead of looking at a series of numbers, you will get a better picture of your progress (Or lack) by turning that jumble of numbers into simple pictures. I charted our data in line graph form because it is easier to see trends on a line. (See Chapter 15, below.)

Your data should be graphed to show the trends for a week, month, quarter, and the year. We followed these procedures during the 18+ years we were in practice. By studying our clinic trends, we were able to predict and correct problems before they knocked on our clinic door. Ask yourself. How can I manage "it" unless "it" can be measured? Surprises are acceptable for a birthday, not a business!

Take Care Of The Big Rocks First!

Your patients must come first in your clinic's operational activities. They are the Big Rocks in the Mason jar of your priorities. Your sole reason for existence is providing patient care. Any situation that hinders that care diminishes your reason for existence!

Taking that idea a step further, differentiate the Big Rocks that are important for your practice. For example, it is usually 20% of your patients who refer 80% of your new business. Or consider your advertising. If you analyze the return on your advertising investment, you'll find that one or two ads result in a disproportionately high return.

Take care of those Big Rocks. Pay extra attention to recognizing and rewarding the special group of patients who refer others to your practice. Consider directing a higher percentage of your budget toward the high-return advertising venues.

I learned about Big Rocks at a seminar when the speaker was illustrating a point about time management. He placed a gallon, wide-mouthed Mason jar on the table in front of our group. He filled the jar with about a dozen fist-sized rocks. When the jar was filled to the top, he asked, "Is this jar full?"

We all answered, "Yes."

He answered, "Wrong!" then proceeded to dump in smaller pieces of gravel. As he shook the jar, the gravel filled in the spaces between the big rocks.

When he asked, "Is the jar full?" Our answer was, "Probably not."

"Good," he said, as he proceeded to pour sand into the jar which then filled up spaces between the rocks and gravel.

He asked again, "Is it full now?" We all shouted, "No!"

He smiled, as he grabbed a pitcher of water, pouring it into the jar filling it to the brim.

Then he said, "What's the point, here?"

Someone raised their hand and said, "No matter how full your schedule, you can always fit some more things into it."

"Wrong," he said. "The point here is if you don't put the Big Rocks in first, you'll never fit them in at all. You must always take care of the Big Rocks first!"

Our patients are the Big Rocks. The way we serve them best is eliminating anything which moves patient care to second place. Your receptionist ignoring a newly-arrived patient to do paperwork is an example of placing patient care second. You can never allow patient service to become secondary.

Phone Interruptions

One of the biggest challenges to a winning practice is the phone. How many times during the day is your patient care interrupted by phone calls? Murphy's Law applies to phone calls. The less you want to be interrupted, the more that phone call is for you!

It usually happens in the middle of an important doctor/patient conversation or adjustment. When you are interrupted by a phone call, the doctor/patient rapport is broken as soon as you leave to answer. When you return, you'll have to spend time re-establishing the interrupted activity. Your patient does not appreciate phone interruptions during their time with you, no matter how important you think it is or makes you look!

If you spend too much of your productive time in phone conversations with loan officers, bank tellers, business development officials, stock brokers, fellow service club members, credit card people, *salesmen,* accountants, bookkeepers, CPAs, tax attorneys, IRS auditors (hope not!), and assorted friends, then set up a filtering system which will control interruptions during patient hours.

Before your day starts, post a call list at the front desk. Your receptionist will only interrupt you if the caller is on your list. If they are not on your list, your receptionist will take a message then you'll return the call later. When I first started this procedure, I would take all calls from doctors, even if they weren't on my list. This stopped when *many* of those doctors were trying to sell me something.

My call list would include:

Expected calls from doctors. When I referred a patient to another doctor (MD or DC) for a second opinion, I found it beneficial to discuss the referring doctor's findings while still fresh in his mind. Many times the doctor and I discussed items not ending up on the final report. However, those notes from our phone conversation enhanced my patient's treatment program.

People difficult to contact during off-hours. Playing phone tag with other busy people was not my favorite activity. Putting difficult-to-contact people on my list precluded excessive call-backs. I did not include social or fellow service club persons on this list. My call-list prerequisite was that the call had to be relevant to clinic operations.

An emergency call from my family. If my wife had been missing a few buttons on her remote control, she wouldn't have been on the list. However, she managed another business and knew that "bring home a head of lettuce calls" were not emergencies. Over the years, the few calls she made were genuine emergencies such as the time she called to tell me our house was on fire and I might want to not to schedule any late appointments.

Carefully restrict your call list, even during non-patient hours. You'll create enough uninterrupted time, even when not seeing patients, to handle the rest of your office chores. Instead of hammering out paperwork after hours, your evenings will be free for community business or social events.

Community Service

The waste of life occasioned by trying to do too many things at once is appalling.
—Orison S. Marden

Remember the old saw: "if you slice the cabbage too thin it's only good for cole slaw." Now that you've established a professional presence in your community, you are being invited to join numerous service organizations. Be selective when deciding which groups to join. Belonging to numerous groups will swamp you with projects. Excessive, non-chiropractic, community activities will negatively affect your practice. It is difficult to manage a practice when your time is being decimated by community projects.

Don't overdo it. There is a fine line between being involved and being excessively involved. Just like a race car going through a high speed turn. You either go through the turn "at speed" or "at excessive speed" *and not make the turn*. You don't want to slide off your goal track. It's's great to be involved in community activities. Just don't become so involved that you are distracted from your primary task, appropriate practice management that benefits your patients.

Our city had excellent organizations such as the Rotary, Lions, Kiwanis, Elks, Moose, JCs, as well as many church and charity organizations. During my early years in practice, I joined everything that moved! My *goal* was to establish a community identity and get involved in some interesting local projects.

Someone must have stopped payment on my reality check, because I seriously exceeded the normal joining process. I found myself committed to too many nightly meetings, countless responsibilities, and an overwhelming number of daily phone messages. Realizing that I had over-committed myself, I changed my community focus.

I reduced my community participation to three groups. This immediately *dropped* my stress level. Cutting back community involvement also greatly improved the balance between my work and play. Lifestyle balance is important. It's an essential element in accomplishing long range goals without burning out.

Write your own "check." Establishing a business in your community also carries the responsibility to volunteer for selected community service. Just writing a check to your favorite charity or local organization *does* not fulfill the definition of community responsibility. You must give some of yourself.

The most expensive "check" a busy person *writes* is for his time. It is a precious and limited asset. "Spend" that check wisely. Investigate a service group before deciding to participate. Make sure the prospective organization reflects your personal service philosophy. Be aware that joining too many organizations will seriously hinder management of your own business and prevent you from doing justice to your volunteer work. It will slow your practice growth.

Say no to "Dougs." I belonged to an organization run one year by a totally committed president. Doug was absolutely focused on doing a good job. He even took that year off work to concentrate on running our club. Doug was a great salesman, so it was hard to say no to Doug when he asked you to be on a committee.

Your ego really gets stroked when someone tells you what a wonderful addition you'll be to their group. Be very careful and remove your ego when deciding to volunteer your time. When you are asked to join a service group or community event, you will be respected if you say no up front. If you're short on time, don't volunteer. Respect for you takes a backslide when you can't do the volunteer work all because you didn't know when to say no to Dougs.

Join for the Right Reasons. Don't get involved in volunteer activities with the intention of boosting your practice unless it's a mutual referral or "tip" organization. Service group members will spot your insincerity. This will erode your community effectiveness and damage your credibility. You must look forward to every meeting. Otherwise, quit, because you're wasting your and the organization's time. Join service groups for the right reasons, to give not take!

Oil and water don't mix! One problem caused by participating in too many organizations is being tempted to do club business instead of practice business *especially during your working hours.* Don't do it! Like oil and water, it won't mix. If you become excessively involved, your fun projects will turn into stressful tasks.. This stress transmits to your patients causing doctor/patient problems. Your anxious state of mind will detract from your primary responsibility, your patients. Be selective, then give 100 per cent of your available time to the group you select!

I received much more from my community activities than I was ever able to contribute. My practice benefitted because participation in my club's activities deepened my people skills. My fellow members had experience levels that were different than mine. By working with them, I learned many things, making my personal and professional life richer. I learned patience, courage, incisiveness, and determination. I also learned from those who were far more committed to accomplishing good than I ever thought was possible. I learned to be a team player. You can't buy that type of experience.

Take a hard look at all the daily interruptions which hinder your clinic and patient services. Evaluate how much time you spend in non-practice activities then volunteer your time selectively and sparingly. Your practice will benefit and prosper.

14

How To Reduce Paperwork Time

You Don't Have to Write *War and Peace!* During my early years in practice, I felt that any report leaving the office was my personal representative. Every report was polished to diamond-like perfection before it was sent out. I was proud of my masterpieces, but I resented the days and nights spent doing paperwork. I discovered that the recipients of my literary gems didn't care if I wrote the greatest novel of all time. All the readers of my paperwork wanted was for the elements their company required to be in my paperwork. All the rest was a waste of words. My originality absolutely didn't count!

I started looking at ways to reduce the time I spent on paperwork. Once I discovered two truisms applicable to all my paperwork, I began to have time for other things.

- Reports and forms for groups such as insurance companies, attorneys, and schools always require the same or similar statements or information.
- The majority of the paperwork can be filled out using common phrases.

Stock Phrases And How To Find Them Make a list all of the paperwork projects now consuming large chunks of your time. Reports to insurance companies, attorneys, schools, team coaches, parents, state and federal agencies, banks, referral doctors, fitness centers, all qualify for your list.

Then look over each project, isolating sections that can be categorized into stock or "boiler plate" phrases. In patient reports, for example, you can use stock phrases that refer to a specific condition. Your patients can either be healthy, have problem(s), or fall somewhere in-between. The various stages all have common elements, so prepare a menu of the possible different patient conditions.

Pick the most applicable condition for your report by just circling its number. If there are multiple reports going to the same place, have several stock phrases available to avoid looking like you stamped them out with a "cookie-cutter."

For example, here is how common elements can be applied to the "Prognosis" section of a narrative report.

Prognosis: (circle the applicable item numbers)

1. Standard orthopedic tests were performed which were essentially negative for pain.

2. Our final examination revealed a satisfactory response to conservative chiropractic treatment.

3. Our final examination revealed pain and discomfort at the injury sites despite conservative chiropractic treatment to diminish the effects of the injury.

4. The results of our final examination directed our conclusion that the patient should expect future episodes of pain as a residual result of their unresolved injuries.

5. Our experience with the treatment of soft tissue injuries leads me to the conclusion that it is probable, even with a current reduction in symptomatology, that adhesions and scar tissue remain in the injured areas. Further I have advised the patient to expect premature degeneration in the injured areas accompanied by localized pain. This pain is expected to exacerbate with stress, physical activity, or weather changes.

6. Conservative chiropractic treatment of this patient has resulted in continual improvement with general symptomatic relief.

Mark your form and kick it out the door!

Multiple choice forms can be created using those and other stock phrases. When designing your forms, make it as easy as possible to select the phrases. The sections pertinent to my reports were checked, additional comments were dictated into a tape recorder, and the form and tape were sent out to a transcription service. I received back a comprehensive report for my review and signature. The transcription expense was a welcome trade for a late night writing reports.

Regular insurance forms can be processed in your office using the same idea of stock phrasing. Your in-house paperwork processing time can be significantly reduced by automation. When I first started this system, I used a word processor keyed to my stock of phrases. With computerization, there are now many software programs to help you knock out the paperwork.

As long as your S.O.A.P. notes can honestly back up your report, the cookie-cutter repetition is irrelevant to the purpose of your report. It doesn't have to be wordy, just accurate. The reader of your report only wants to know the status of your patient. Give your reader the information they're looking for and you're done with your report.

Bank forms can be handled creatively, too. When dealing with a bank, even on a short term basis, you usually have to fill out long, tedious forms. The way I handled those bureaucratic beauties was to make a copy of the completed form. Whenever my bank needed an update, if there was no new information, I just changed the date on the original and re-submitted. If there was new information, I added it to a copy of the original completed form as an addendum.

The only time this procedure changed was when the bank changed forms. I then simply repeated my original routine.

An Alternative Method

Another way to reduce your paperwork time is to train a staff member to do your reports. The staffer completes your forms using your notes from patient's charts. This staff member must be trained to interpret your chart notes. Then, he or she must be capable of translating those notes to your report forms. Remember, for best results, choose a staff member that understands your philosophy of report writing including your writing style.

You will have to invest some time into training the selected staffer so that when you put down your notes, the staffer can use them to choose the proper pre-constructed phrases on your reporting forms.

Your notes, either coded or paraphrased, will guide your staffer in assembling your report. Your report preparation time is now reduced to review, adding in a few special comments, and signing the report. So, instead of spending your nights staring at piles of undone paperwork, create an automatic reporting system.

You won't need much equipment. The resources needed to produce reports can range from paper and pencil to a staff dedicated to that one job. Your goal, when producing a report, is to spend as little time and money as possible during the process. Treating patients adds to your income stream not reports! This means get someone else to do most of the work and obtain just enough equipment to do the job. Over the years, I used several types of equipment to produce my reports. I also used tape recorders to customize existing phrases.

There are easier (and more costly) ways of producing reports. I have observed my colleagues complete their reports right after they see their patients with the use of expensive, special equipment. If your volume warrants the expense, hand-held computer systems can greatly speed up the reporting process. After recording your exam and treatment protocols on a special hand-held computer, you can then download it into your main computer. A staff member can then generate a complete report from the downloaded information. Hand-held computers are useful. These allow you to dictate and download directly into your main computer, bypassing all other humans. There are even software systems enabling you to dictate your report directly into *your* main computer.

The fact that you have room in your budget to buy the latest report-writing equipment doesn't mean you should run out and buy it before you investigate it thoroughly. This may not be an easy task, because every product will claim to be the best thing since Wonder Bread built your strong body. You will be better off to visit a colleague who has been using the software or equipment you are considering. Talk to someone who has been using it for a while, not to the ad executive who spent his time figuring out ways of convincing you to buy it.

George Carlin once observed, "I noticed that a box of croutons proudly exclaimed they were packed in an air-tight envelope. Why bother? They're just stale bread!"

Another method is to use a tape recorder. Talk to the recorder during your patient's visit, then turn in the tape for transcription. That's it! When the hard copy crosses your desk, just review and sign it. However you input your data, once it is entered, your work is done! Move onto more productive tasks.

When you're less involved in the paperwork-producing business, you'll appreciate being able to leave the office with a clear conscience. Your unfinished work won't be flying around your head like pigeons waiting to drop a message saying, "don't leave until your report is finished!"

If you keep in mind, when determining how to accomplish your paperwork, that your goal is to identify tasks that can be automated, delegated, or eliminated, you can pay more attention to tasks that only you can perform as The Doctor.

When prosperity comes, do not use all of it.
—Confucius

15

Cash Flow

Rich or poor, it's good to have money.

Money, in the form of cash, is a prime indicator of a the health of a business. Conversely, the vast majority of small business failures come from a single cause, poor cash management.

This is a strong statement. It means careless tracking of money flow will result in serious complications. Simply put, without the life-blood of cash, your practice will die! Your appointment book may be full, patients may be coming and going, you're running every minute of your day, yet if your cash flow is marginal, you're almost out of business!

Profits and Cash Flow In 1997, according to Sutton Landry, Director of the Small Business Development Center at Northern Kentucky University, "69 per cent of all U.S. business had annual gross revenues of less than $50,000. 78 per cent had annual gross revenues of less than $100,000. These are virtually identical percentages to a decade earlier....Given the kind of static revenue that most small businesses are generating, it is little surprise that two-thirds of all new businesses fail within five years and most surviving small businesses don't even show a profit for three to five years."

Landry concluded that the road to solving cash flow problems was to avoid getting in debt through borrowing, raising money by selling assets, or implementing similar weak solutions. Cash flow problems are best resolved by getting to the root of the problem, which is almost always a lack of profitability.

Among chiropractors, cash flow problems can usually be traced to operational weaknesses.

Chiropractors typically experience cash flow problems if:

- The collections department is unaware of their job responsibilities or is just goofing off. This can be happening at either the front desk or in the billing area.
- They spend too much on expenses that can be controlled. Many of these costs may be non-essential to current operations.
- They make payments on equipment (postage meters, rehab equipment and, yes, even x-ray equipment) that produces minimal or no profit.
- They have excessive or non-producing office space. The huge office may satisfy the ego, but it can be even harder on the cash flow.
- They tie their cash up in excessive inventory such as vitamins, pillows, supports, or X-ray film.

How many of these conditions describe your practice? Do you know where your money is coming from and where it is going? Do you know your current financial condition and where it is heading? Up, down sideways? Perhaps it's time to start watching your cash flow!

Unless you plan for the normal ebb and flow of your cash supply, a catastrophe may lurk right around the corner. The only thing that saved me, the one time I got careless with my cash flow early in my career, was my financial trend charts.

I used two methods to follow my cash flow, cash-flow projections and charts of my financial trends.

Cash-flow Projections

You can construct a simple projection or make it very complex. It depends on the time and energy you want to invest. The more details, the better the forecast. Whether it is bare-boned or highly detailed, a cash projection is a must!

Balance sheets and Income / Expense reports that you can construct yourself or obtain from your CPA can provide you with excellent insights into whether the money flow is a river or a stream. They also inform you where money is being used and in what quantities, and they pinpoint the areas that you might want to modify.

The projection I used was fairly simple. I derived income and expense figures from the income statement provided by my CPA. I added in as many variables as I could determine. This ranged from how much I might borrow for personal use, how long it takes to collect money from insurance billings to vacation times for myself and patients, holiday distractions, and any predictable advertising or marketing expenses.

These figures were plotted out as far as I felt was accurate. As each plotted time period was reached, I entered the actual figures and compared them to my estimates. If there were major differences, I adjusted my future cash flow estimates. After several months, a fairly accurate picture of my cash flow and anticipated cash needs started to form.

The chart on the next page illustrates a three-month period.

Interpreting The Cash Flow Projection

Looking at the anticipated figures for January, you can see where I missed the boat in several areas:

- Income was overestimated by $6,650 (Some patients didn't pay!)
- Refunds were more than anticipated.
- Office Supplies were overspent by $50 (Not too bad!)
- Salary was higher than anticipated because of my personal needs. (Broke my race car)
- Payroll taxes were revised upward by my CPA due to changes in tax planning.
- Credit card expenditures were double the estimate. (Just had to go to that seminar!)

As a result, my income was lower and my expenses were higher than anticipated.

I had anticipated a final January cash balance of $14,600 when, in actuality, it turned out to be $4,200. Now, what do we do? We adjust next month's anticipated figures.

We anticipated February's income at $20,500 due after discovering our that collections department hadn't done its job. We tuned up the collections department, knowing income would increase as a result. I also increased the other items in the February anticipated column to match the actual figures from January.

"In the "Let's See If We Need More Cash Section," I then took the Final Cash Balance figure of $4,200 and posted it in February's "Cash To Start The Month column.

Alas, my hopes for better collections during February didn't work out. We had mistakenly counted our money before it was collected and committed to a strong advertising program ($2,500). Although everything else was on target, those two miscalculations resulted in our having to borrow $2,000 to cover February's expenses.

In order to determine what March held for us, I also posted, in the "March Projected" column, $11,000 in anticipated fees. I also decided to take $1,000 less in salary for March.

Delman Chiropractic Cash Flow Forecast

	Jan. Real	Jan Prob	Feb Real	Feb Prob	Mar Real	Mar Prob
Income						
Pt Fees	18,350	25,000	11,000	21,500		11,000
Ret/Allow	1,000	500	1,000	1,000		1,000
Tot Inc.	17,350	24,500	10,000	20,500		10,000
Expenses						
Advert.	500	500	2,500	500		2,500
Equip Lease	1,250	1,250	1,300	1,300		1,300
Off Supp	200	150	300	200		300
Rent	2,500	2,500	2,500	2,500		2,500
Salaries	6,500	5,000	6,500	6,500		5,500
Tax/Pyroll	2,200	1,000	1,200	2,200		1,200
Cr. Cards	1,000	500	1,000	1,000		1,000
Total Expenses	14,150	10,900	15,300	14,200		13,300

Let's See If We Need More Cash Section

Cash to start the month	1,000	1,000	4,200	14,600		20,900
Income	17,350	24,500	10,000	20,500		10,000
Expenses	14,150	10,900	15,300	14,200		13,300
Cash Bal.	4,200	14,600	(1,100)	20,900		17,600
Needed Cash	0	0	2,000	0		0

After adding in the $2,000 for February, we had $900 left over to start March. We anticipated that we would still be $2,400 shy of making our expenses for March, therefore I also anticipated that I would have to find yet another $3,000 to cover expenses for the month of March.

Don't be put off by all the figures. After doing this several months, it'll only take you a few minutes each month to do the projection. The benefits of this monthly exercise could be the difference between failure or survival of your practice!

Plan for the unexpected. Consider adding an additional 10% to your anticipated expenses for the unanticipated expenses. You will not be sorry!

My first CPA didn't like my projection. He said, "It isn't quite up to proper accounting form." It made sense to me, however. I used this projection (or some form of it) for over eighteen years. My practice prospered and grew. That's good enough for me! Check it out. See for yourself.

Why You Should Chart Statistics

When I first started in practice, I had no visual systems to monitor my current financial condition or the direction of any trends. I was running a race without instruments and *wouldn't* know if *I* was *in* trouble until the motor broke! Of the many seminars I attended, two were very helpful in demonstrating how to graphically depict financial status. Sterling Management's "Management By Statistics" and Greg Stanley's "Whitehall Management Seminars."

After attending those two seminars, I started a system of statistical management. Those simple systems are still being used by the doctors who took over my practice. Like the gauges in your car, they are only valuable when they are utilized! And just like those gauges, all they do is indicate a potential problem. You must take an action for its resolution!

Around my fifth or sixth year, our statistical trends set off a warning buzzer. They indicated, though our office was well-booked with patients, that the differential between services and collections was continuing to increase. I found, to my amazement, that billing was not high on my staff's priority list. After a meeting reminding the collections group their sole purpose is to collect monies owed to our clinic for services already rendered, the trend reversed and a cash flow problem was averted.

During that period of time, I realized that an important component to being aware of the financial direction of our practice were graphs of our statistics. Be aware, however, it's like having just one napkin when eating ribs it's helpful but not enough! The doctor must have a more comprehensive understanding of his practice's finances than just trends. He must have financial plans for taxes, savings, investments, equipment, times of low income, and so on. Some of those items were beyond my capabilities at the time, so I started looking for help. After talking to many local business people regarding their recommendations, I eventually hired a CPA. I gratefully unloaded all my financial data in his office. He also convinced me to have all my clinic checks written by a local bookkeeper. All I had to do, then, was review and sign them. In essence, I was taken out of my clinic's financial management loop. That was a big mistake!

A year later, my practice was in worse financial chaos than when it bumbled along without all that "expert" help. This experience taught me an important lesson. I had to learn how to interpret financial data so I could better analyze the figures and their meanings.

Start By Asking Questions

A prudent question is one-half of wisdom.
—Francis Bacon

After looking over the smoking financial ruins left by my last financial "advisor," I hired a new CPA. This time, I changed a few procedures. I started writing expense checks myself. This forced me to review every expense generated by my practice. At first, considering my work load, I thought it was stupid to stay late at night reviewing bills and writing checks. I soon learned, however, that it was not stupid, just time-consuming. It was also time well-invested. After a month or so of doing this, I started to see a more detailed picture of expenses that my statistical trends had failed to address. I was also fortunate that one of the CPAs in my new firm had the patience to answer my financially uneducated questions. During this period of time, I got a crash course in basic, operating finances.

By now, I had some idea of how my money flowed. This, coupled with the trend graphs, enabled me to avoid crashing on the Reef of Low Cash Flow during the slow months.

With a CPA firm feeding me information regarding when and how much to pay on taxes plus giving me quarterly data, I now had the financial facts necessary to properly run my practice.

There are many sets of numbers that flow through your business: patient visits, appointment data, new patients, collections, and so on. Instead of flooding my desk with an overwhelming amount of numbers, I picked four or five which would give me a balanced picture of my operations at any point in time.

Numbers shotgunned across a page do not personally show me as good a picture of what they represent as does a graph. I prefer the line graph for displaying data. Line graphs provide me two types of information: 1) Current status of that statistic and 2) The direction those numbers say they are heading.

By knowing the direction your practice is going, you'll have "early warning" signals of impending problems. Solutions are much easier to apply early in the life of a problematic situation.

Your statistics and graphs are only as good as your data-gathering procedures so be as accurate, as possible. Also, remember that a "normal" trend is upward, not level.

Charting Practice Trends

My interest is in the future because I am going to spend the rest of my life there.
——Charles F. Kettering

There are numerous ways to chart practice trends. There also are many different sets of figures which can be used to plot clinic trend lines. (Pick the figure that you feel gives the best picture of your practice direction in concert with your goals.) A statistical overview of our operations coupled with a review of our financial statements provided excellent, up-to-date pictures of our clinic's activities.

Below is the process I use to develop my charts. It is not the only way, however. If you have never constructed charts, start here then modify the procedure later to fit the needs of your practice.

Line Graph Basics: Before we get into chart construction, here's a quick refresher on making and interpreting a line graph.

A line graph displays a trend. A trend is a statistically significant change in performance data. The direction of the data performance is measured and illustrated by the graph.

A line graph is a way to summarize how two pieces of information are related and how they vary depending on one another. The numbering along the sides of the graph is called the scale. Labeling the graph, as simple as it sounds, is very important. Otherwise you'll have two lines without the reader knowing what they represent!

In our line graph there are two axes: The vertical axis is called the Y axis; it represents *position*. Position are units of any type of performance data, such as number of patients, fees collected, etc. The horizontal axis is called the X axis; it represents *time*, such as months, years, etc.

When both axes are laid out, it will look like an "L." The finished line graph will be a picture of your performance over time. The direction a line travels on the graph shows a trend, or a statistical change in performance over a given time period.

Before you start plotting your data, find the range of your data then make certain all your numbers will fit on the page.

There are three basic points to remember when you are plotting your data:

- There must be at least three points of data on your chart before you can determine even the start of a trend.
- When the horizontal (X, or time) axis is plotted too close together, there will be excessive vertical (Y, or performance) swings To keep this from happening, plot your data further apart.
- Weekly data swings are informative; however they don't give you a clear picture of your trend. I recommend plotting monthly data points which will give you a better trend picture.

How To Build Your Charts The process of developing your chart starts with collecting accurate figures and posting them onto a spreadsheet. Those figures are the ones which will be plotted on your chart.

I used four data fields: New Patients, Total Visits, Services, and Collections.

Month	New Patients	Total Visits	Services	Collections
Jan	18	1050	51823	38328
Feb	14	930	43354	24283
cumulative	32	1980	95178	62611
Mar	20	1027	50060	29210
cumulative	52	3007	145238	91821
Apr	21	1133	53581	34209
cumulative	73	4140	198819	126030
May	31	967	47453	26380
cumulative	104	5107	246272	152410
Jun	22	1009	42441	26773
cumulative	126	6116	288217	179183

Exhibit A: **Data Summary - January thru June**

Exhibit A (above) is an example of a data summary sheet showing the first six months of the calendar year for the above four data sets. The numbers for our graph are taken from this sheet then plotted onto the charts. The first example is Exhibit B: New Patients, below.

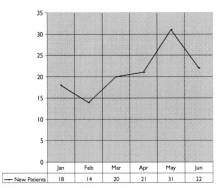

Exhibit B: New Patients

With the New Patient numbers plotted on the chart for the first six months of the year, you can see this is a moderately strong upward trend. If this practice can keep up this trend, it will be in good shape regarding new patients by the end of their calendar year.

This chart also informs you of the rate of new patient increase. If the rate is unsatisfactory, action can be implemented to increase the positive angle of the new patient curve.(In this case, I would be satisfied with this rate of increase. Some offices I have seen would have problems servicing a huge influx of new patients over a short period of time. It is better to have a steady increase and "fine tune" the operating protocols of your practice as you handle the new patient volumes.)

As you start constructing the various charts, keep in mind they are interrelated. One statistic has an influence upon the other. Look at all the data contained in all charts as parts comprising your total statistical picture. The numbers and graphs, when properly interpreted, will describe your practice status at that point in time.

Now, let's look at a chart depicting Total Patient Visits (Exhibit C, below). Observe the flat trend line (it is interpreted as a negative trend). There is a blockage somewhere in the system of this practice!

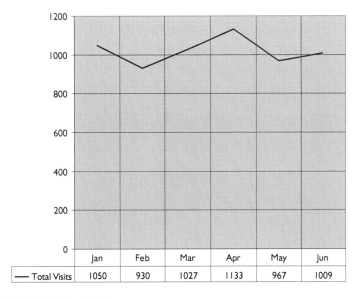

Exhibit C: Total Patient Visits

Earlier, we noted the New Patient chart was on a strong upward trend. The neutral direction of the Total Patient visits trend possibly may be related to the way patients are handled after the initiation of their treatment protocols, because when new patients are taken into a practice and patient retention procedures are followed, there should be a higher number of patient visits.

The best way to analyze the source of a blockage is to check over all aspects of a practice in detail. Until you do, any number of explanations is possible; each needs to be examined. The causes could be anything from an inability (or unwillingness) of the Front Desk to handle an increased patient volume to the doctor subconsciously not wanting to increase his work load. Despite the "gray area" nature of the analysis, the chart has handed you a starting point to investigate the problem's causation and eventual correction rather than by guesswork.

There were several walls we bounced into during our time in practice. These all caused problems we had to correct:

- I spent too much time talking to each patient about subjects not related to their treatment.
- There was insufficient staff follow up regarding patient scheduling despite information noted on the treatment card.
- If a follow up date was noted, the Front Desk failed to confirm it with the patient.
- Our first visit fees were excessive for the area.
- Our office hours were inconsistent making it difficult for the patient to know when we were open to take care of them.

That gave us a start on where to investigate.

Look at the chart of Services (Exhibit D, below) for our sample practice. As noted earlier, there is a relationship between the various data bases, therefore, it is best to look at them all when looking at the entire data picture.

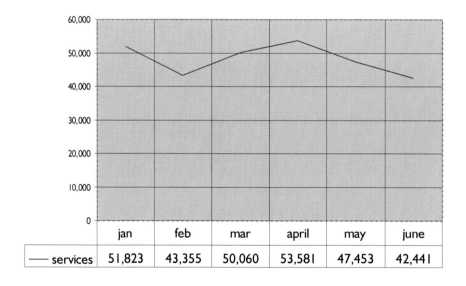

	jan	feb	mar	april	may	june
services	51,823	43,355	50,060	53,581	47,453	42,441

Exhibit D: Services

As you look over the chart, you will notice a decline in Services for the three months of April, May, and June. Remember, to determine the existence of a trend, there must be three points of reference. In this case, the decline in service fees probably relates back to the neutral (negative) trend of Total Patient Visits.

Again, this chart gave us an area to investigate rather than our having to guess why our incoming dollars were in decline.

Another useful chart is one where Services and Collections are plotted on the same sheet (see Exhibit E, below).

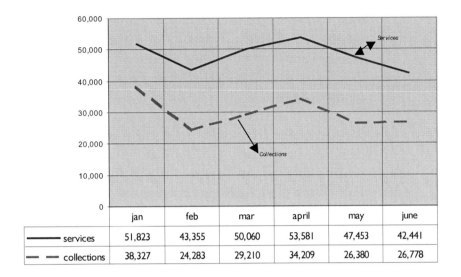

Exhibit E: Services and Collections

I put these two data bases together so you can look at their differential. Note the gap between Services and Collections. That is the magnitude of your receivables (the fees you have not yet collected)!

Ideally, these lines should run closer together. In the real world they sometimes do not. In fact, there are times when these two graphs become reversed This happens when your collections are catching up to your services. If you have been running behind on collections for a sustained period of time, a surge of incoming late collections will cause the Collections graph to cross over Services and run above it. Normally, Collections will lag slightly behind Services unless you have a total cash practice.

Taking a hard look at the Services / Collections graph pinpointed areas where we looked for corrections. Here are some weaknesses I found then corrected in our collections area:

- The patient was not initially informed of his financial responsibilities.
- The Front Desk personnel had problems asking patients for payment(whether co-pay or cash fees).
- The Collections personnel were inconsistent with their billing cycles.
- The Collections personnel did not understand their primary task was collections!
- I was weak in my management of the collections group.

Start With These Numbers

During my years in practice, the four main statistics I constantly monitored were Services, Collections, New Patients, and Total Patient Visits. (Substitute any other statistics you feel important to monitoring your practice) I plotted my statistics for the week, the month, and the year. I was not too concerned over the results of the weekly graphs. I would not start looking very closely until we had graphs for a month. At that time, I would start incremental changes in my operations.

At the three month level, I expected to see positive results from those changes. I would again make changes if the graphs were trending in the wrong direction after three months. The yearly graphs showed me how well the team had achieved our goals and helped me plan for the next calendar year.

Graphing results and coupling that information with cash flow forecasting resulted in a strong practice, no matter the condition of the economy. The sooner you start monitoring your statistics, the sooner you can take control of your practice rather than letting outside economic influences take control of you.

Question Constantly, Change Cautiously.
—The Author

16

Your Management Style

The Big Picture

Just like a painter working on a mural, you must occasional step back and get an overview of your total practice. When you do, you should ask several questions:

- What areas of my practice do I have to strengthen to make it stronger overall?
- What strategic planning will I have to formulate to compete in the current changing marketplace?
- What changes in my practice will I have to make to keep it growing?
- What further education will I need to enhance my practice growth?

This questioning should be a continual process. The core element for maintaining a strong practice is an ongoing evaluation through consistently asking yourself and staff questions. This enables you to react to changing business conditions. Questioning is an essential element in keeping your practice growing and healthy.

Get Off Your Duff and Manage!

It is not the crook in modern business that we fear but the honest man who does not know what he is doing.
—Owen D. Young

At one time or another, we all have had problems with the way our office functions. The methods which we use to solve these problems widely differ, but none can be successful unless the end result is a return to your operating guidelines. This may sound simplistic. But the fact remainst that the simple details we ignore are the ones that grow into difficulties. This is well illustrated by a front office problem we were experiencing.

When I first started in practice, all my time was spent learning my craft. Most startup problems were easily handled except at the front desk and insurance areas. I reasoned that the back office was working out better because I was mainly in that area during patient hours. When there was a glitch, it was easily spotted and quickly resolved.

The front desk and insurance areas were a different story. I incorrectly assumed that the staff members who had prior experience in those areas would know how to perform their jobs with minimal supervision. When the declining numbers in their departments were brought to their attention, I also incorrectly assumed that the problem would be dealt with in an appropriate manner. The two departments had so many different functions that I always found excuses not to learn the *basic* details of that area. As their statistics declined, I realized something positive had to be done. That's when I started, Mobile Management.

Mobile Management, as discussed earlier, is simply setting aside time, every day, to walk around the entire office to observe all procedures. If I didn't understand something, I asked. This accomplished several objectives. I eventually got a pretty good understanding of all office operations and my staff knew they had to have the answers to what they were doing. This gave me the impetus to learn the basics of all office operations, first by observation, then, when time permitted, by performing the job itself. This covered all staff-operated positions in the clinic. Knowing the basics of each job enabled me to better evaluate the capability of each staff member to deal with their responsibilities.

Better educated, I instituted modifications that strengthened our office procedures. We began to see positive changes.

There were times, however, when some front office employees either refused or were unable to comprehend what was expected of them Despite admonitions, goal meetings, and re-training, there was no other recourse left but termination. This was a last resort decision when all others measures failed.

As manager, you must take time to understand the functions of all your office operations and utilize that knowledge to further the goals of your mission. As your practice progresses, train several staff members who understand your goals to do the staff training.

Remember the Big Picture. That doesn't mean you have to do it all, but you must be able to recognize when a function is not operating up to your standards and then to correct it. The best way to keep tabs on a clinic is to know how it all functions. Get out from behind your desk! Observe how your office is operating. Spending

Looking for the Tip of the Iceberg

Short as life is, we make it still shorter by the careless waste of time.
—Victor Hugo

your valuable time to obtain this knowledge is a wise investment in the future of your practice.

Being busy doesn't justify dropping your level of service. Do you become disturbed when you enter a treatment room and your patient starts in on you about how long they had to sit in *your* "Waiting Room"? You should because it's your responsibility!

As your practice gets busier, there are more distractions to prevent you from getting your patients through the treatment process in a reasonable time. Your staff pushes you to move along, because they are the ones fielding complaints and don't appreciate the flak.

Your busy practice pulls at you from several directions and you start feeling more pressure. You find yourself "pushing" patients through your procedures. Perhaps you start taking short cuts in your exams. As the pressure increases, your standards start slipping.

The patient who consistently sits too long in your "Waiting Room" becomes less compliant. Eventually, you lose those patients when they find an office where they can obtain satisfactory treatment that respects their personal schedule.

For every patient who tells us about a problem they have with our practice, there are many more who say nothing. I used to drive staff wacky whenever that happened. Sometimes they would attempt to downgrade the seriousness of the complaint by saying, "Oh, Mr So-And-So is not a happy person with anything." My answer was we absolutely had to investigate all complaints. "It's the tip of the iceberg," I would say as the staff grimaced from that frequently-repeated answer. "There are patients out there not complaining. We'll lose them if we don't investigate!"

The excessive patient waiting problem usually was caused by scheduling new patients too close to regular patient hours. I was consistently late by using up regular patient time for new patients. We were able to rectify that problem at subsequent staff meetings.

As our patient volume increased, other problems caused by operational weaknesses would surface. The causes would quickly be identified and eliminated before they got out of hand. There was a time when I handed out the supplements and explained usage recommendations to the patient. I know the patient appreciated the explanations; however, those conversations put us behind with our patients. This also happened with dispensing appliances and similar items. It is important for a patient to understand why they are getting a supplement or appliance and how to use them properly, but there had to be a more efficient way to deal with this situation.

We decided to do three things:

- We handed out pre-printed sheets with the same explanatory information we previously verbalized.
- We trained the back office person to have a good working knowledge of the items we dispensed to patients. That person was also responsible for the inventory. Her inventory responsibilities gave her an excellent opportunity to read the literature on those items. After we had discussed the recommended usages of our inventory items, she was able to answer most of the repetitive questions posed by our patients.
- We set up a consultation or obtained additional literature for a patient requiring more detailed information.

By following these procedures, our patients received acceptable answers. We had identified, then removed, the obstructions to a smooth patient flow.

Spend a few minutes, after hours, to list the tasks that take a lot of your time. Then see if you can either delegate the repetitive portions to your staff or streamline your part. This will allow your patients and your staff to better plan their time. Your "Waiting Room" will then become a true Reception Area.

Are You Listening?

If I have ever made any valuable discoveries, it has been owing more to patient attention, than to any other talent.
—Isaac Newton

A race car driver listens constantly. He listens when tuning a motor. He listens to his crew chief and spotters during a race. He listens, with trepidation, to every little mechanical sound during the last laps of his race. He listens!

Once of the big gripes I have had since childhood is that many people don't seem to listen. They are either too busy preparing their next comment or, when you are speaking to them, they're either interrupting or are somewhere on planet Mars. Don't you hate it when you're talking to someone at a gathering and, instead of looking you in the eye, the clod keeps looking over your shoulder wondering who else is at the party? In political circles that's called "working the party." I think it should be called "working on being insensitive."

Non-listening is so commonplace, I have learned to watch people's eyes. When they start to glaze over or even worse, roll up into their skull, it's my signal to stop talking. I then ask my benumbed listener a question in order to wake them up. I try to do fewer pontifical monologues, and I think I'm getting better because I've been asking fewer questions lately.

There are many ways to hold a listener's attention. Some are drastic, some more subtle. "Silence is one of the great arts of conversation," is a great statement, illustrating a valuable tool. To focus attention on your conversation, just stop talking. It usually works.

Another attention-holder is to change your voice volume. Raise or lower it. At times, I'll do something more drastic and gently touch that person to get their attention just a touch, especially if they're holding a full glass. It's considered rude with possible legal ramifications to do much more.

Do Your Patients Fall Asleep During the ROF?

When giving a Report of Findings to your patient, consider their state of mind. A patient can be distracted by their pain or a long ROF. Perhaps they are an "A" personality who just can't sit still very long. Since informing your patient is so important, plan how to give that information for maximum effectiveness.

I'm aware that soap box seminars can be boring to a semi-interested listener, so I offer my information in planned segments. My initial ROF is short and to-the-point. Each time the patient comes in for treatment, they are given another segment of their report. This has worked for me. Any method that gets your patient to understand what you are saying will work as well. The key is to acquire, then hold on to, your patient's attention while you communicate information to them.

Don't give up on your ROF just because your dozing patients are falling off their seat. Maybe you're droning on and on and on about a point that could be made more succinct. Try your ROF on an honest friend and see if they get your message. If not, it's time to revise your ROF.

There is no way you'll be able to educate your patients if they don't listen to you. Your staff must also be aware of this fact. Their own conversations with patients must effectively reinforce your message. They, too, must be sensitive to the patient; so if they are talking to a patient and start seeing only the whites of their eyes, it's time for them to change the subject, too.

I received my most effective communications training by participating as a member of Kiwanis and, later, Rotary. When you are a guest speaker, the members will be polite. When you are a member of that club giving a report or announcing an event, unless you make it attention-getting, you'll feel like Rodney Dangerfield. No respect! Participation in a service organization is great for developing effective communication skills.

On Being Polite

Life is not so short but that there is always time for courtesy.
—Ralph Waldo Emerson

It is our obligation to treat patients with courtesy. We all know that. Yet, we occasionally fail in that task, some practices more than others. There are times when we'll get busy and forget we're in the service business. Who do we service? People!

Being courteous to your patients is a basic component of a successful practice. All of us have experienced discourteous treatment from people whose job was to provide personal service! We've all heard countless horror stories regarding someone's visit to another doctor's office. Now, that same person was in our office, telling us about someone else! Your practice should not function like the one that chased this patient away!

The first impression of your office, whether by telephone or in person, happens at your front desk. If there is disservice at the front desk, the negative ripple effect will hurt your practice. Reversing the damage is much harder than preventing its occurrence.

Sometimes the disservice is subtle. For example, a patient is kept waiting at the front desk while your receptionist yaks away on the phone. Train your front desk personnel to place a caller on hold until the waiting patient's needs are handled.

Another subtle discourtesy is a sliding glass door at the front desk. Don't you love it when you tap on the window, it slides open, the person tells you to sign in and then closes the glass doors in your face! As you impatiently wait, the office staff on the other side of the closed glass doors are having a Roman party. And you keep looking at your watch! If you are remodeling, you should consider an open reception area.

I'm Managing Everything!

As a manager, be careful not to micro-manage. Getting involved with minutiae will eat up all your time. Your responsibility is the big picture. If the task at hand can be delegated, do so. Provide guidelines for the completion of that task. As a concerned manager, it is easy to over-control the operation of your practice. This creates unnecessary work and results in functional problems. Constricted management creates bottle necks in the decision-making process because no one has the final authority except yourself. This is not good business practice. Be careful not to trip on the details as you lead the charge to your goals.

Bend or Break

Things do not change, we do.
—Henry David Thoreau

Always remain flexible in your thinking.

Prior to becoming a chiropractor, I worked as another kind of adjustor—in the insurance industry. After a period of time working outside, I was "promoted" into management. I discovered that things in the office did not always work in a straight line.

The company I worked for was huge. It had its own ways it wanted us to perform our office tasks and routines. These were dictated from corporate headquarters, which was only a little closer than Mars. It was bad enough that the procedures didn't always translate well to our field office. What made it worse, for me, was the fact that every quarter the company sent new instructions it thought would improve operations.

I went crazy every time the new protocols arrived. Just as I was getting comfortable with one system, a new one came along. I was expected to embrace it and then convince my field personnel to make it work. When each installment of "improvements" arrived, my manager listened to me rant about the changes that had just rolled down from corporate Mount Olympus as I waved the new paperwork in the air like an alligator waves its prey.

During one of my temper tantrums, my boss took me aside and introduced me to the wisdom of flexibility. He taught me that I could better manage the garbage that came down the corporate slope if I bent with it rather than fought it and that the energy I wasted fighting the system could be better used to implement the latest program du jour. He helped me understand that being a strong manager does not mean being so strong and stiff that you break.

This one principle more than any other helped me get through the "my way or the highway" period of my young management life. By opening the door to my previously closed mind, I could see that the bureaucratic pronouncements from Corporate Mountain occasionally contained good ideas.

Manage your practice with the same open-mindedness. Be flexible enough to recognize worthy staff suggestions, for example. Consider their suggestions even if you have to modify your original plan. Not only will you get along better with your staff, you won't find yourself dropping concrete blocks of dictatorial ideas on their heads.

Teamwork or Tomahawk? You and your team must share the desire to move your practice in the same direction. A team is strong when it pulls in one direction and wastes its strengths when it pulls in different directions. You probably know what happened when a committee was formed to design a horse—they ended up designing a camel. If your team isn't functioning on the same page, then they'll end up throwing tomahawks into your management machinery or designing camels.

"Me talk, you listen" doesn't work. To get the results you desire, you can't just tell all the staff where to go (although at times that might be tempting). It is important to involve everyone in the planning, operation, and goals of your practice. That's the best way to build a team that will help to raise your practice to the accomplishments you seek.

Directing Your Staff

As a manager, your task is to conceptualize, initiate, then achieve. *You* are supposed to control and direct your practice. If *you* don't, ask yourself, "Who does?" You'd be surprised at the number of clinics where the tail wags the dog. How many times have you seen an office where the staff really runs the show? Perhaps subtly, but still in control. In most cases, their goals, no matter how virtuous, will not be the same as the doctor.

Is it wrong to have a strong staff? Heck no! It's an asset! You just want them to go in the same direction as your mission since it's also their mission. Their guidelines must emanate from management.

Although control of your clinic's direction comes from you, staff input is essential. Your decisions must be consistent with the goals of your clinic. If your staff is acting on ideas that are inconsistent with your goals, they must be re-evaluated and/or re-trained regarding their understanding of your mission and goals.

Your task, as a manager is to motivate and educate your staff so they accept and work toward your vision by implementing your goals. The direction of your clinic will either just muddle along or head toward your staff's version of its destination.

Your practice is a reflection of your dreams. It is, after all is said and done, your vision.

We're Too Busy for New Patients?

It is not enough to be busy; so are the ants. The question is: What are we busy about?
—Henry David Thoreau

During one of our weekly staff meetings, we all were reviewing the statistics and graphs for the previous month. We noticed our new-patient statistics were on a downtrend. Discussing the situation at the meeting provided no specific answers.

In order to see if there was a "situation" (same thing as problem but sounds neater) at the front desk, I observed how staff handled their areas of responsibility. The front desk staff seemed to be doing a great job following our operating guidelines. One day, while I walked by the front desk, I heard a new staffer tell a caller we were too busy to see them that day. I almost choked! I had the staffer recall that person and get them in that day.

Our policy was if we couldn't fit in a non-scheduled patient during normal office hours, then we'd stay late to see that person. All new employees were asked before they were hired if staying late presented any problems. If so, they couldn't be hired.

Apparently, that new front desk person didn't like to stay late. She didn't want to tell me she wanted to go home after regular hours, so she arranged the office schedule to suit her own purpose!

The problem was corrected with new personnel at the front desk. Our new patient statistics returned to a normal condition shortly thereafter.

A chiropractic practice becomes strong by the consistent application of conscientious patient service which is guided by your office policy regarding patient management. That's one more place where staff meetings serve a good purpose.

Conversely, a front desk that operates outside of your policies will destroy your practice. (A graph showing new patient intake will give you warning before the other shoe drops.)

Working Hard versus Working Smart

How many times have you been told, "You must not just work hard; you must also work smart?" Having heard that saying more than I want to remember, I said, "Heck, it could never apply to me. I know what I'm doing!" I ran my clinic with that poor attitude until our growth came to a grinding halt.

No matter how hard we all worked, it was a chore to see more than 35 patients during regular business hours. Our office always seemed to be staying open *after normal hours* to make certain everyone was seen. I felt if I tried to speed up, the quality of my service would decrease.

I checked with some colleagues; they were seeing more patients during the same amount of time! Their techniques and office protocols were similar to ours, so I was stumped. Then I attended a Greg Stanley practice management seminar.

After the seminar, I cornered Greg and discussed my problem. It took him five minutes to come up with the answer. He said that my clinic had two discernable barriers to patient flow. First, I talked too much. Second, the way patients moved through actually held my practice back.

Both were inefficient procedures and obstructions to further growth. He drew a recommended change to my office layout on a napkin and left me standing there in amazement.

Monday, I excitedly returned to the clinic and started changing operating procedures. We all tried to keep patient conversations limited to chiropractic subjects. If the patients needed more time, we asked the front desk to set aside time for an uninterrupted conversation. Few patients wanted the extra time.

Most of the patients felt their questions were just socializing and did not want to "take up more of my office time." The few patients who opted for the extra time were able to have a private conversation which was better for both of us. Within 30 days, we sailed past our 35 patient plateau with little effort. We didn't have to change our office hours, and patients appreciated being able to get their treatments within the limits of their own busy schedules.

The items Greg pointed out were basic and obvious. I didn't recognize them because we were not working very smart. I also realized my head was buried in the minutiae of running my clinic. This prevented the necessary planning which would have identified the problem and solution Greg illustrated on that seminar napkin.

From that time on, we started staying after the clinic closed to evaluate our day's work, plan for the next day, and see if any improvements could be made in our operations. The total time spent each day, after seeing patients, probably averaged an hour. Pick a time fitting your disposition, early morning or later at night. As your clinic matures, that extra hour will return big dividends in clinic productivity.

Alternative Plans Just in Case

Among mortals second thoughts are wisest.
—Euripides

When racing, you always have contingency plans. At all the places where you might overrun the track, you pick out an escape route or *a similar alternative.* At all the places where you might have a chance to pass another car, you figure alternate ways to make the pass, sometimes on the inside line and sometimes on the outside. The same principle applies to the management of your practice.

Always have a "Plan B," or alternative plan, ready to implement, just in case. The process of establishing a contingency plan will prod you into evaluating your current clinic status. The operative words here are planning and flexibility.

It is to your advantage to be in a position to change your mind, change the way you operate your clinic, or at least listen to another opinion. When you make plans, don't set them in concrete. If you are inflexible, that concrete will drag you down the bottom of Lake Failure. Be ready to modify your plans, as needed.

The concept of adaptability extends across all the operational lines of your clinic. For example, we realized a common barrier to bringing in new patients is excessive first visit fees. We found that when we lowered our fees to a "break-even" level on the first visit, several things occurred.

- The number of new patients increased.
- The increase in new patients offset the decrease of income from our lower first visit fees.
- By emphasizing education, we retained enough new patients to increase our total practice.
- We automatically developed a market niche for our clinic. In a small town, the word spreads rapidly when there is a good "deal" for potential patients.

We received feedback from a few colleagues who said we were trying to start a "fee war" or something like that. Some of our staff were concerned with that reaction, but subsequent practice statistics corroborated our decision. If our decision to lower fees was not in line with our goals, our statistics would have dropped. We would have then reversed our decision and tried an alternate plan.

The decision, which resulted in lowering the financial barriers to new patients, was clear and proper in light of our mission: "To positively affect the health of our community." A flexible attitude will allow you to make positive changes to practice operations.

In order for you to serve and prosper, your organization and its mission must be the foremost consideration in the decision-making process. A vibrant, growing practice best serves its community.

A man always has two reasons for doing anything—a good reason and the real reason.

–J. P. Morgan

17

Diagnosing Your Practice By Priority

In order to move your practice to a higher level, you must recognize and eliminate the barriers to advancement. Have you ever thought about diagnosing your practice and its procedures as you would a patient? I know when my race car needed a pre-race checkup, I would approach the car checkup the same as a patient examination. By systematically examining my car, asking questions, and observing carefully, I collected enough data to form a diagnosis that helped me plan my course of action.

Whether you're analyzing a race car or the functions of your practice, the approach is the same. Prioritize *your* areas of investigation according to importance, then challenge or examine them in a systematic, questioning manner.

For example, suppose your practice is low on cash and you cannot meet all your monthly payments. Your diagnosis is, "Hypomobile Cash Flow." How do you examine the situation, triage the areas of concern, arrive at a diagnosis, and then proceed with corrective action?

If you try a "shotgun" or "do-a-little-for-everybody" approach to paying your bills, it will not be as effective as taking a more focused approach. A focused approach starts with preparing a list of all the payments due. Then, you examine the entire list prioritizing the items you absolutely must pay versus the payments which can be deferred. As a courtesy and to keep friendly with your creditors, call all those whom you are deferring and explain the short-cash situation. Most will understand and appreciate your call. You then make your payments each month according to your prioritized list, stopping when you reach the limits of available cash.

How about reducing expenses on a more nearly permanent basis? An excellent preventive course of action is to examine each expense area and determine its significance regarding its contribution to the life of your practice. For instance, when you are going over the list and notice seminars, travel, or entertainment are at significant levels, curtail expenditures in those areas. When you can satisfy such items as rent, taxes, and other contractual items, then consider easing the lid on your elective expenses.

There's no magic here. Still, you'd be shocked off your hi-lo tables to see the many doctors who completely miss this point! Every month they run out of cash, yet they continue to spend until they are so deep in a financial pit that climbing out is almost impossible.

Here are a few more items to consider when you have to reduce your practice expenses:

Evaluate your facility. Too many offices have unproductive space. Evaluate your space in terms of what it produces for your practice. For example, reception areas are unproductive. X-ray rooms are partially productive and busy adjusting spaces are very productive.

Look at your storage areas (they're unproductive) in terms of the cost of that space. Would it cost you less if you rented nearby space outside your office? If you are stuck with excessive office space, consider renting that space to a complementary profession such as a psychologist, podiatrist, or family therapist. You'll recoup some of the money you're losing on that square footage.

I once built a monument to my ego. It had been a large, stand-alone bank building. The remodeled building was beautiful. I was impressed, my patients were impressed and my community was impressed. It was a wrong move! After I filled that palace with enough staff to move patients, additional doctors to make the space productive, and communications systems to cover all that space, I had enough left over to buy myself a pair of roller skates to help me cover my areas of management. I realized my net had been better as a solo practitioner. I sold the building and reopened as a solo practitioner in a smaller facility. I learned a practice can be stronger and more fun when it's not competing with a big overhead.

A solo practice needs only about 1,000 square feet in which to operate. The trend away from private adjusting rooms requires even less space for a clinic facility.

Evaluate your outside services. Ask yourself if the film processor must be cleaned as often. Does it have to run all day? Could the office be cleaned by your own personnel? Usually this can be addressed at the staff meeting. The choices could be as simple as wage reduction vs. staff cleaning. Do you have coffee or similar services? Even as a temporary measure, reducing these services slows down your cash bleeding. When you again develop discretionary cash reserves, you can re-institute some of the reduced services. This, again, can be brought up at the staff meeting. Give your staff a list of services and ask them to make choices. It's a win-win deal.

Survey your equipment service contracts. How often do you need maintenance on your equipment? If there's a breakdown, how much is it to fix versus the contract cost? For example, most copy machine service contracts don't cover one of the most expensive of repairs, the drum. A cost-benefit analysis might surprise you! Many times, you'll find your equipment does very well without service contracts.

Review employee perks. Travel expenses, company cars, entertainment, staff seminar expenses, all should all scrutinized. Are they necessary for the daily operation of your practice? If you must travel, shop for the best buys. There are companies that can save you hundreds of dollars on airline tickets, for example. The same applies to hotels and restaurants. If you absolutely must attend that miracle technique seminar, ask yourself the following questions:

- What person(s) must absolutely attend this seminar?
- Can the person going to the seminar teach those who don't attend?
- Is this seminar really necessary, or is this an excuse for a vacation?

Even if the "clinic" is paying for all expenses, remember, that "clinic" is you!

Review utilities and other equipment.. How much are you spending on heating, air conditioning, and lighting? On the days when you have only staff in the office, turn the lights on only in working areas. Air conditioning use should also be minimized. Some managers even place locked covers on the control boxes to prevent expensive yo-yo temperature adjusting.

Telephones can cause significant losses to a practice. Examine your billings and ask the phone company for their free analysis of your call patterns. If getting a handle on excessive, out-going phone calls is important, certain telephones can be setup only for incoming calls. The phones capable of out-going calls can be assigned to specific personnel.

The same thinking can be applied to on-line computer systems, faxes, and copy machines. All can be controlled if their costs of operation are getting out of hand.

Consider your contributions and subscriptions. Belonging to a service club is a monetary as well as personal commitment. Can you afford it? A temporary leave of absence will ease the burden of the club's dues and costly service obligations. Taking a temporary leave keeps the option open for your return when your money situation improves.

Service to your community through an organization is an excellent activity, but be aware that community service doesn't directly contribute to your income stream. In fact, when you are struggling with your practice, service club activities will dilute the time and effort you could be dedicating toward making your practice viable. Service club members want to have you volunteer to help them. That's the nature of a service organization, However, first take care of your business, then take care of your community.

When examining your practice, start from the head (you) and move on down. It is more effective to examine one area at a time before you move on to the next rather than to attempt to look at several problematic regions simultaneously. Unless you have a large organization, I recommend that you become aware of how each level functions in every area of your clinic. You and no one else should do the examination!

18

Retaining Patients

Are you happy with your patient retention? You should be. You spent years learning how to be the best chiropractor you can be. You've spent or you will spend additional years building your practice. You've invested a lot of time and money to get each patient who lies on your table. It's a lot easier and a lot more effective to keep that patient than it is to find a new one.

Remember, you aren't the only Chiropractor in Dodge. You work in a competitive atmosphere. There are always hands who think they are faster than yours and want a piece of your action. What is it that keeps your patients coming to you instead of going to the saloon down the street? It is not your technical skills, as prodigious as they might be. It is you and the service you provide. Your task is to make your hands special, to be remembered, and to justify your patients' loyalty.

You *could* lower your prices, but then your competitors could match your generosity and where would you be then? The better way is to make your services special and valuable to your patients. They don't come to you because you are the only one who can help them with their problems. They come to you because of who you are and the relationship they have with you.

How many one-time patients have you seen over the years? You probably bent over backwards to ease their pains. Why didn't they return? Some of them might say "money." That's a different issue. Many of them may answer, "Your treatment was fine, but I prefer Dr.

Jones down the street." Why Dr. Jones? Because he has developed a stronger doctor/patient relationship with them than you did.

I sold my practice in 1995. When recently re-visiting my old town, I saw former patients on the street or in a store. Many of them said they wished I was back in practice. Some were just being polite, however, the rest were saying they missed my service They didn't miss my technique, shiny equipment or explanations of the subluxation complex. They missed our relationship.

The Doctor/Patient Relationship

Building good doctor/patient relationships begins when you build your practice around the perceived needs and desires of your current and prospective patients. Examine those patient's needs and desires. You'll discover they're more interested in trusting relationships, personalized service, and relief from their presenting condition than they are in your years of study, current techniques, or shiny new office.

When you're talking with your patient, relate your discussion to your patient's situation and use examples such as, "John, if we can get your shoulder to be more functional, it should improve the smoothness of your golf swing." Or, "Frank, I know the G-forces in turn nine are creating a lot of neck pain during your race. If we change the shape of your head rest and apply some chiropractic treatments, we should be able to reduce the strain and get your neck to work more naturally. Then you'll be able to better focus on your race."

Scratch That Niche!

Another way to better conceptualize and communicate the benefits of your service is to place it into a special category. Get across to your listener that you are special, that you understand their situation, and that you have been successful in solving the problem they are presenting to you.

Dr. Sharon excitedly emailed me recently with an idea that worked very well for her. She had been reading our booklet, "111 Tips for Managing a Profitable Chiropractic Practice" when she came across the tip about enhancing your practice by developing a specified market niche.

Dr. Sharon thought about that concept. She had been a cheer leader in high school and college, so she knew the special physical stresses cheer leaders experience when they practice and perform their routines.

She contacting her former cheer leader buddies and coaches. After several months of phone calls, her work started to pay off in visits from her friends and inquiries from the coaches. Some of those visitors turned into patients after they realized Dr. Sharon had first-hand knowledge of their injuries and residual damages and that she had the training to help them return to a better physical condition.

Dr. Sharon continues to build a practice that is interesting and exciting. Her practice is also starting to provide the financial returns she needs to be able to continue her excellent service. Every one wins, because Dr. Sharon created a team of her patients and herself. They know that she cares and that their goals are the same.

Create a niche for yourself, like Dr. Sharon did. It will allow you to focus your attention on the particular demands of that particular niche. This allows you to become an expert where an expert is needed and to concentrate your efforts where they will be appreciated.

Watch Your Language

Another way to build customer loyalty is to speak with your patients, not at them. Don't just use words. Produce pictures in their minds.

When you tell a patient you want to give them a "Checkup," does your patient understand what you're trying to communicate? Or, do you have to throw words upon words to explain what you mean? Instead of saying, "I want to perform a spinal checkup on you," for example, try saying something like, "Let's find out how that damaged area we worked on last time is moving and functioning." The word, "checkup," isn't a visual word. It doesn't paint a picture. Yet, people visualize pictures better than abstract word forms. If your goal is to communicate an idea, placing a picture in your patient's mind is a powerful way to do that.

Words set the tone of a conversation and determine its outcome. Do you tell patients that you are "recalling" them or inviting them in for a "necessary periodic re-examination?"

Listening is a mutual activity. Listen to, don't just hear, what your patients are saying to you. People often speak with more than words. By listening carefully to what they are saying with all your senses, you will know what they are thinking. Does your patient tell you, "Hey Doc, I just need an adjustment of my sixth cervical." If so, the patient is telling you that they are in charge of their chiropractic treatment and you're just another wrench in their tool box.

You are the doctor. You, not they, must remain in charge of their chiropractic care. Perform whatever work you feel is professionally correct before the requested adjustment. By doing this, you illustrate three important things to the patient: You don't take the administration of their care lightly; you respect their body;

therefore, in return, they need to respect your expertise. At the same time, remember that your patients have valid concerns. You need to listen to them, too. This is a partnership and a dance, not a tug of war.

Involve Your Patients

Listen, or your tongue will make you deaf.
—Native American proverb

Your patients must feel that they can rely on you for professional chiropractic services. More than that, they need to feel that they are valued and important. They have to feel that they are participating with you and not simply being worked on by you, that they are players, not cash cows.

You are preparing your patients for a life-time of wellness care. The best time to do this is when they tell you how much better they feel and how much they admire you as their guru of wellness. You have just established a rapport with your patients. Now is the time to talk with them about taking care of their entire body and not just adjusting their neck.

Impress on your patients that the body is not static like Stone Mountain, which has remained unchanged for years. Communicate the idea that the adjustments they have just received are parts of a life-enhancing mechanism that requires periodic maintenance. Emphasize the concept of pay now or pay later. By neglecting well-being now, patients will pay a lot more later, not just in time and money, but also in unnecessary suffering.

Why do you want to get your stabilized patients on a scheduled appointment as opposed to a drop-in-when-you-feel-like-it basis? Because this is the beginning of a commitment. If the decision to return is up to your patients, the commitment falls very low on their priority list. You lose control and turn into an unused tool sitting in the box waiting for your patients to determine the status of their own health.

A week or so before their appointment, contact your patients and either confirm or have them call you to confirm. The idea behind this, once again, is to involve the patient in the appointment process and strengthen their commitment.

Involve your staff. Your patients interact with them at least as much as they interact with you. Get your staff on the same road as you. Make sure your staff knows what you expect and how to help you achieve it. The behavior and attitude of your staff are some of the main factors that make a visit to your office a pleasant experience. And the patients' experience in the office is one of the reasons why they come back or go elsewhere.

Get Feedback Happy patients seldom leave. Try to find out what your patients think of you and the work you do. Don't wait until you start getting requests from one of your local colleagues for a patient's records.

Most of your current patients probably like you. They don't want to hurt your feelings. When you ask them how they like the treatment you are giving them, they may well tell you that you're a fabulous chiropractor and that they don't know what they'd do if you didn't practice there any longer. What many of them tell you, however, is what they think you want to hear. Unless you are really sharp at reading body language, interpreting neurolinguistic clues, listening to the tone of voice, or watching eyes, you may not spot any well intentioned dissembling.

Many chiropractors find that the best way to get honest answers from patients is not to ask the questions themselves. Instead, they hire third parties to obtain information about their practice and the value of their services. Marketing research clearly reveals that people will give more nearly honest answers to a third party than to a interested party. The independent survey may not give you the answers you hoped to hear, but it will give you the data you *need* to ensure that you retain your patients.

Once again, listen to what your patients really tell you. It is the only way you can evaluate whether your services measure up to what your patients want. We all need constant feedback. Even if you end up referring a client or two to a colleague, you will still have made the point that you do respond. That's a message they will not forget.

The use of money is all the advantage there is in having it.
–Benjamin Franklin
(So don't tie it up in inventory.
–The author)

19

Inventory Control

Is Your Practice An Inventory Smithsonian? As a business owner, one of your jobs is to determine the usage and turnover of your inventories. How long do your supplements stay on the shelves? How often is a patient dispensed a pillow or some other appliance?

Once you determine your turnovers, you can set minimums and maximums for your inventories. Actual inventories can then be listed on a sheet (See Exhibit F, page 110) and staff can then physically handle the actual ordering, stocking, and so on. You deal with it only if your inventory stocking parameters are changed.

Another of your jobs is to evaluate your equipment usage. How productive is your equipment? If you have a dinosaur taking up space in your office, either make that ancient, unused equipment earn its keep or get rid of it! Donate it to a needy colleague, a charity, your school, or the museum, but get rid of it! Dusty machinery is a distraction and takes up space. Utilize the space vacated by the unused equipment *more* productively. Some experts call it "efficacious space utilization." I call it smart!

If you have equipment, it must be maintained. Even the simplest hydrocollators need cleaning with stainless steel cleaners on the outside and element cleaners on the inside. If equipment requires maintenance, which is a cost both in time and material, then that equipment must be productive to justify that maintenance expenditure.

INVENTORY CONTROL TAKEN JUNE 30							
Item	In Stock	Hi/Lo Level	Vendor	Phone Number	Quant. Order	Date Order	Date Rec'd
Vitamin Z	3	3/7	Backdoor Sales Co.	333-4800	3	6/30	
CryoPaks	15	3/15	Penguin Co.	444-Cold	0	—	—
Knee Brace	2	2/6	Pretty Patella, Inc.	378-5600	4	6/30	
Cerv. Pillows	6	5/10	Lordosis, Ltd	434-7700	4	6/30	
Copy paper	3 reams	4/10	Cellulose Corp.	536-Tree	7	6/30	
Pencils	12 boxes	1/3 boxes	Mr Slick Pencil Co.	478-2100	re-evaluate	—	—

Exhibit F: Sample Inventory Control Form

Do you purchase every pretty brochure you see, or do you have a theme or plan? Look hard at the office literature you have in your office. Do you have stacks of literature shotgunned all over your office? Does the literature reflect your practice philosophy? Is there anything stated in the literature that might cause your clinic embarrassment?

I've talked to doctors who have been skewered in court due to some piece of literature obtained from their own office. The literature's text was *taken*, usually out of context, to embarrass the doctor and diminish the impact of his testimony.

Ask yourself a few questions about the published material in your office:

- Does it help educate your patient in the subjects you want them to know?
- Does it help promote patient referrals?
- Is it well presented in your reception area? Does it occupy a special place?

- Do you have literature in your treatment rooms so you can personally hand it to a patient at the appropriate time?
- Is your literature just gathering dust?
- Does the literature contain any claims or statements that will embarrass you, your clinic, or your profession?

A room with an overabundance of literature is distracting to your patients who just see a lot of "stuff." A smaller selection would have greater impact and make selection easier for the potential reader. Specific literature in each adjusting room is a powerful tool and a great time saver in a busy office. A note made in the chart regarding the dispensed literature will remind you to ask the patient about it on the next visit.

How to Reduce the Cost of Inventory

In everything the middle course is best; all things in excess bring trouble.
—Plautus

It's easy to figure out how much money is tied up in your inventory (just add it up) but have you ever figured out how much time you invest whenever you have to explain a dispensed product? Having supplements and appliances on your premises is handy, but is it economical for you to dispense them personally? Having an inventory and dispensing vitamins to patients is not necessarily cost-effective. Our most cost-effective work is adjusting patients.

Assess your vitamin and appliance inventory. You'll find hundreds of dollars tied up on your shelves. You'll also find certain supplements are "gathering dust" on your shelves as they are shoved aside by the "Product of the Month." Reduce your inventory to items not available locally and return what you can for credit. Check your suppliers to determine how long it takes from order placement to the receipt of various items. This will allow you to reduce carried inventory and, in effect, to let your supplier do the stocking.

Go out into the community to shop supplement stores and find a quality referral source. Choose one where the owner takes the time to explain their products, an owner who stays on top of the nutrition industry and carries quality products at a fair price. Refer your patients to the store you choose so the owner, not you, can spend time educating your patient. Don't worry about getting referrals from the vitamin store. Your purpose is to make certain your patients have access to quality items accompanied *by* educated explanations.

Evaluate everything X-ray film, office supplies, literature, and so on. Trim, upgrade, or dispose of excess quantities of those items.

Types Of Inventory

There are numerous methods to control inventory. The three most common are:

Perpetual Inventory. This method maintains a continuous tally of items purchased or sold. The tally can be kept either manually or through a tie-in with a computerized system such as transaction registers. This is expensive and, unless your practice sells and maintains a large inventory, I do not recommend it.

Selected Inventory. This method involves determining which items of your inventory have the greatest volume of sales. Usually the categories are divided into three or four control sections. The higher the volume, the greater the control of that item you should exercise. This system fits the needs of the small practitioner. The key to the success of this program is to accurately determine the applicable control categories for your inventory. When this is established, you then apply the least formal controls on the lowest volume items and the most stringent controls on the highest volume items.

Visual Inventory. This is the method most used by doctor's offices. This system is the most successful for the solo and small practitioner's office. The key to making certain this system works is to have a dependable staff member who performs periodic visual inventories. One person must be responsible for the frequent assessment of the inventory. That person must also know the lead times necessary for replenishment of the items in the inventory. We utilized this type of system and experienced few problems.

Using the Visual Inventory System, a simple form is made up which lists all of the inventory items. The following information is needed on the inventory form:

- Item description
- Current inventory level
- Hi / Lo levels. The "Lo" level is determined by the lead time necessary to receive an order after placement. The "Hi" level is determined by the turnover speed of that item.
- Vendor name and phone number.
- Quantity ordered.
- Date ordered.
- Date Received.

The criteria for order size is also based upon discounting, monthly specials, minimum order quantities and cost of the items.

Occasionally, you should audit the inventory levels and purchases. However, if the person in charge of watching the inventory stays within your guidelines, your inventory will remain at reasonable, cost-effective levels.

The inventory person is responsible for going through new catalogs to note best buys or to spot new items for discussion at one of the staff meetings This person is also responsible for checking incoming orders for proper items received and correct count. This system ties up a minimal amount of money in inventory, catches shipping mistakes and keeps you up-to-date on possible new items for your office. The added responsibility will strengthen your staff members' commitment to being part of your team.

> *Harmony of aim, not identity of conclusion, is the secret of sympathetic life.*
> —Ralph Waldo Emerson

20

Personnel Matters

The Importance of Harmony

The elements of a successful practice are many. An enthusiastic, optimistic practice is composed of a multitude of synergistic details. One of the most important details is harmony.

Harmony is synonymous with peace. You have to be at peace with yourself and your surroundings before you can dream and grow.

Peaceful does not mean complacent. If your statistics indicate you are on a plateau, you might be experiencing a complacency which can hinder your personal growth as well as your practice.

If you want to grow so you can better serve your community, you and your team should be in agreement with your mission and its goals. You and your team must consistently, persistently, and harmoniously push past any barriers toward the next level of your practice.

Harmony also implies symmetry, or, stated another way, consistency and reliability in agreement with order. Your team has to pull the practice equally. If an engine is out of balance, it runs terribly. If your team is out of balance, your practice either slows down or the other team members have to work asymmetrically in order to accomplish your projected goals. That unbalanced situation eventually deteriorates. Below are a few examples of practice disharmony. If any of these rings a bell, then perhaps you might want to take a few steps back to obtain a clearer picture of your clinic's daily operations.

You might have "practice disharmony" if you:

• Have patients in the reception area who have been waiting increasingly longer times before you see them (Watch for muted mumbling!)
• Fail to follow up with the patient on a recommended home treatment.(After too long a period, when the patient is finally asked, he says, "Huh?")
• Are not reminded to call the new patient to see how they are doing after their first adjustment. (On the next visit, the patient tells you repeatedly how much they suffered because they didn't know about ice packs)
• Treat a member of your team with favoritism over another. (You start wondering why your staff turnover is increasing)
• Discipline one staff member out of proportion to the others.
• Have patients set their own appointment schedules and ignore your recommendations (Your patient visit graph goes into decline).

Work at getting all of your staff and all of your patients in harmony with your mission and goals. Some patients will fall through your fingers and some staff members will not necessarily be in accordance with your thinking. Losing either those patients or employees who are "not in sync" with your team will not hurt your practice. As long as your clinic progresses in a reasonable direction and functions as a single-purpose unit, it will operate much more smoothly.

In summary, if you don't consistently press forward as a unified, harmonious team in agreement toward one goal, it is a given that you will definitely stumble backward in disunity.

Your Safety Belt: Your Staff

Trust [your staff] and they will be true to you; treat them greatly and they will show themselves great.
—Ralph Waldo Emerson (amended)

You must have a strong staff to lean on! You don't develop a strong staff by accident. It requires planning, then execution. You are the teacher providing, whatever education and direction is needed from your staff.

Our dedication, as chiropractors, is in the service of the people. As doctors, by definition, an important portion of that service is education. The initial group of people who must receive the benefit of that education is your staff.

Your staff must feel part of your organization so their goals will be the same as yours. If your staff accepts your vision and goals, then, when you have to alter course, they will understand and help you re-direct the focus of your practice.

A simple step often overlooked is defining who the top management person is in the clinic. One of the costlier management misjudgements we have seen made is having a wife or girlfriend (husband or boyfriend) function in a management position. If you have to hire your wife (girlfriend, whatever) to staff your office, then that situation should be limited to six months or less. Someone that close to your personal life can wreck your staff and office operations. It is the exception rather than the rule when a husband/wife combination works well in any business environment.

One of the problems with a husband/wife combination is that the staff and later the patients become confused as to who is in charge of managing the clinic, the doctor or his wife. This creates confusion and seriously hinders the growth of the office. Two bosses with different agendas will destroy your team! If you leave this situation in place for any extended period of time, correcting it'll be costly and emotionally traumatic!

The other day, I was grocery shopping and observed the store (one of a large chain) was noticeably cleaner, better organized, and better stocked than its sister stores. All of the employees we met were friendly, helpful, and more knowledgeable than in other stores. Many of the details and displays throughout the store showed much thought and creativity.

We were so pleased, we complimented one of the department supervisors. She immediately pointed to a man standing in an aisle checking some shelves. She told me that man was the manager. He is the person who guides them all in how they set up their store. I realized this person knew what he was doing. His staff was involved. All knew his vision for his store and they were proud to help him work toward that vision. The efficient yet friendly demeanor of that store was proof he was getting his message across.

When you give a staff member authority for an area, be careful not to dilute that authority. Follow the proper rules of management. Give that person a clear picture of what you expect from them with guidelines on how to accomplish your expectations. Hold that supervisor to your requirements but do not bypass his authority by micro-management.

We all, at one time or another, have subverted the rules of departmental authority. Who among us is not guilty of walking a patient up to the front desk, bypassing the receptionist, and making a new appointment for that patient. That's micro-management! All of this while the receptionist was available for the same task. Unless the front desk is so overloaded it affects quality patient service, allow the receptionist do their job! When you bypass a staff member, it de-motivates their future work performance.

Hey! Aunt Millie! Want a Job? When you are first starting out in practice staffing is usually a reaction to an immediate need. Hiring activities are sometimes not well thought out. Staff members in new practices are often installed like

> *The employer generally gets the employees he deserves.*
> —Walter Gilbey

cheap decals on a window, with similar results. Some stick, some fall off, and most barely hang on! Just like the decals, all of them look great before application. Many times that new hire is one of your new patients, a neighbor, or (gasp) even a relative.

The abilities and contributions of your staff should mature and grow along with your practice. During the time I was in practice, mistakes were made when hiring staff. Those mistakes were noted and an effort was made to not repeat them. After many hires, a pattern started to take shape. This pattern guided my future employment practices.

For the first ten years of our practice, I had more personnel turnover than a flapjack festival. After being hit on the head by the 2 x 4 of turnover enough times, I woke up and realized there were good reasons *behind* both our good and bad personnel choices. It became apparent to me that the qualities of a prospective employee's personality are more important than their work experience.

During the early years of hiring, I searched for people with prior experience in a chiropractic or medical office. That didn't work out! The applicants were usually poorly trained in effective office procedures. My office seemed to be a magnet for applicants who possessed the personality of either a turnip or an alligator! This was especially true for applicants with prior experience limited to a medical office. The way they dealt with patients absolutely did not fit into our operating plan. I concluded personality, life experience, and demeanor were the major factors to look for in job applicants.

I also discovered several criteria *which are* important when evaluating applicants for staff positions. An applicant would tend to be more successful adapting to our office procedures if they:

- Were a current or past chiropractic patient. The chiropractic experience is unique and is best understood as a patient. This knowledge is valuable when working with other patients.
- Had minimal, or preferably, no medical office experience. Most applicants who had medical office backgrounds appeared to lack rapport with the patients. Staff members with prior medical office experience "handled" patients in a less personal manner than those with work experience in a chiropractic practice.
- Were a mother with teenage children or had experience in the care of children. The emotional roller coaster environment of raising children develops the compassionate sensitivity needed for dealing successfully with patients in a health care environment.
- Were capable of juggling several tasks simultaneously. This included the ability to smile and greet patients, note their arrival

in the appointment book, and pull their chart, all while having the phone glued to one ear answering a caller's questions.

Once we found a person who fulfilled a majority of the above requirements, training them about the details of the position was an easy task. The exceptions were insurance personnel, who should have prior billing and collection experience.

Staff Meetings: Monologue or Dialogue?

Half the world is composed of people who have something to say and can't, and the other half who have nothing to say and keep on saying it.
—Robert Frost

A review of SBA case studies confirms that many employees don't know what's expected of them. This indicates poor management communication that can lead to inferior job performances by employees. An excellent way to open the portals of communications between management and staff is two-way meetings in which both management and staff become involved in the discussion.

Webster defines dialogue as "a conversation between two or more persons" and "an exchange of ideas and opinions." This definition describes an ideal staff meeting. In our staff meetings, we expected and encouraged everyone to provide input.

On the other side of the spectrum, a monologue is defined as "a long speech monopolizing conversation." Does that describe your staff meeting? Does everyone have input or are there just a few who take over the meeting and pontificate?

For a busy office, a consistent policy of having staff meetings is sometimes difficult to maintain. Time constraints tug at you to cancel "just this one meeting" which then leads to further cancellations, and so on. Don't fall into that trap! Staff meetings are not for show. They're for two-way communications!

If your staff meeting is a format to show how powerful the management hierarchy is, it is not performing its function. I have seen staff meetings where management sounds like they belong on a pulpit or in a locker room. There was no exchange of ideas. There was no volunteering of information from the staff. When your staff is silent during a meeting, there is a shortage of trust between management and personnel. You're not communicating, and that will damage your practice!

Staff meetings serve several important purposes. They:

- Establish communication between staff & management.
- Share the current operating status of your office.
- Discuss solutions to operational problems.
- Plan new objectives toward goals.
- Plan new goals when the old ones are attained.
- Establish a common purpose for the practice.

A staff meeting should have an agenda. Your staff should have that agenda prior to the meeting. This allows time for them to prepare their thoughts and comments. Reviewing prior weeks statistics, successes, failures, discussing barriers to achieving goals, future plans, or changes in goals are all worthwhile subjects for staff meetings. Complaints about other staff members or perceived inequities should not be discussed in the staff meeting. These are personal matters and should be discussed privately with management.

Since time is important, getting too far off course from the agenda is non-productive. The meetings should not drag. I found that sixty minutes each week was sufficient to meet all agenda items.

A timely, productive meeting requires a moderator. The doctor has to be this moderator. He has to cover all pertinent items and still keep within the planned time.

If you have a multi-doctor clinic, you should still should designate one doctor to run the meeting. At the beginning, it is a good idea to name a different doctor each meeting so you can evaluate who can best run an efficient, productive staff meeting. That same doctor should also be chosen as the liaison between staff and management between meetings.

Staff meetings are not social hours. They are the time to resolve barriers to goals and reinforce common objectives.

The Need To Know

Employees want and need to know the full scope of their jobs. They also need to be informed about your practice goals, new operations, and the problems you need to resolve. Your job is to communicate this information to your staff.

The basic kinds of information your staff need to know are as follows:

- What they are expected to accomplish on their job? This is where job descriptions come in handy. Have the person who has been doing the job write the initial job description." Then, sit down with the employee and edit that draft to your specs. This will save you, the busy doctor, from the hassle of writing up all the jobs in your office from scratch and autocratically expecting employees to march in lockstep..

How will they be trained for their job?

- The blueprint you'll use to guide the training of your new employee is the job description. Whatever is essential to performing the job can be extracted from the job description and made into a checklist that can be used as a training outline. Delegate training new employees to one of your staff. You'll have a much better chance of ending up with a thoroughly trained new employee by using this easy method.

Training new employees for your practice is as important as training a new driver in the rules of the road. You don't want your employees to be like Henry, who, when asked about the difference between a flashing red light and a flashing yellow light answered, "the color." You can be a passenger in his car if you want. I'll walk. Imagine how your patients would react if they met Henry behind your front desk.

Your employees will have their own questions. Make sure they know the answers to things like:

- When will I be eligible for any vacation time?
- How many days of vacation time will I accumulate with job seniority?
- Are there any incentive or bonus plans?
- How do I qualify for bonus or incentive plans?
- If I qualify, what amount of money is involved?
- What holidays and other days will we be closed?
- Will I be paid for holidays and closed days?

In addition to information about their immediate jobs, your staff should understand and be able to explain to others basic information about the following areas:

- The techniques and therapies you are currently using in your practice. Over the years, I used several types of adjusting techniques. I didn't expect my employees to know about these in detail, but I did advised my staff that they should call it the "Gentle Delman Technique" when they were discussing methods of adjustment. I assured them that I would provide a more detailed picture when I consulted with the patient myself.
- Any vitamins or ortho supplies that are part of the inventory, especially new items.
- Techniques and therapies that you are contemplating adding to your practice.
- Changes in the patient flow or work area modifications. I once planned to modify the flow of patients in my office. When I shared my idea at the staff meeting, one of them pointed out a basic flaw in my plan. By discussing the changes before we implemented them, we saved a lot of wasted time, money, and aggravation.

In addition, it is important to keep employees informed about matters affecting your practice such as:

- Your performance statistics. Post your basic performance graphs in an area where they can be seen only by your staff. Then, discuss them at your weekly meetings.

• Changes in your outside environment (such as new laws), changes in vendor status (such as financial difficulties), and new practices within your marketing area.

• Changes to the information contained in our personnel manual. Once a year, the person who designed our personnel manual updated it. We had one meeting with her to a discuss these changes.

Employees want to know about their company, and more importantly, matters affecting them. Keeping your staff informed goes a long way toward satisfying that requirement.

There are three main ways you can communicate the above information to your employees: weekly staff meetings, the personnel manual, and the staff bulletin board. A fourth, less formal channel, is gossip. You cannot regulate gossip. All you can do is be certain that whatever you tell one employee is fit to be learned by the others.

Policy Manuals

Give me the [policy manual] rather than the ready tongue.
—Giuseppe Garibaldi (amended)

One of the keys to developing a strong and productive staff is to have in place methods which will guide them toward solving the problems they will encounter in their areas of responsibility. For example, if you have a meeting with an employee regarding a problem and that problem is not resolved, that problem now becomes yours! The staff member must leave a meeting with directions on how *they* can solve the problem. A comprehensive policy manual is an essential tool for helping your team resolve their office policy questions.

The manager who tells an employee, "I'll get back to you on that problem," and doesn't, de-motivates that employee. Somewhere down the road, that manager is going to get blind-sided by his employee's problem. Guidelines that are clearly stated in a comprehensive policy manual, become excellent tools for dealing with most personnel questions.

A policy manual is an easy way to communicate the complex rules under which business is required to function. In these days of governmental involvement in our business affairs, care has to be taken not to expose your practice to unnecessary legal complications brought on by failure to adhere to some obtuse governmental regulation.

The best way to put together a legal yet understandable company policy manual is to hire a labor expert. Be wary of software programs or "fill-in-the-blanks" policy manuals. Those "by-the-number" systems are inadequate. You need to keep current with rapidly changing regulations that constantly flow out of state and federal governments. An annual review of your manual by one who works in labor relations is the best way to go. The cost, when amortized over the year and compared to the cost of the personnel problems it resolves, is reasonable.

I was fortunate to know someone who worked for a large aerospace company and was very knowledgeable in this area. She also was in process of developing her expertise into a full-time career. This expert compiled an excellent policy manual and updated it once a year. It was an excellent investment. Even if she had not been available, we would have found another competent personnel expert to handle the job of building the manual and keeping it current.

When we received the completed manual, all our employees were required to read it (on company time, in a quiet place). They were then asked to sign a sheet indicating they had read and understood it. If there were questions that more than one staff member raised regarding the manual, we brought up those questions in the next available staff meeting.

A copy was always available for any staff member to look at. If a policy question was brought up by a staff member, they were referred to the manual. This saved me a lot of time answering questions about sick days, vacations, and so forth. If the manual did not clearly answer their problem, we called our consultant for clarification. If a particular section failed to address the needs of our clinic, our consultant made the appropriate changes to update our manual.

Topics Covered in a Good Manual

Consultants typically charge a flat fee for putting together a policy manual plus an annual fee for updating it. There are usually no fees charged for questions during the year or for any changes made to clarify wording. To better illustrate the depth of a professionally prepared policy manual, here is a list of topics covered in Delman Chiropractic's manual:

- General statements
- Reporting of absence
- Attendance
- Bereavement leave
- Progressive discipline
- Dress code
- Employee classifications
- Employee notification of policy changes
- Employee records
- Employment of relatives
- Garnishments
- Holiday benefits

- License verification
- Medical leave of absence
- Military leave of absence
- Overtime-non-exempt personnel
- Pay advances
- Payroll check distribution
- Personal leave
- Reference requests
- Rest and meal breaks
- Review Program
- Sexual harassment
- Sick leave
- Solicitation and distribution of literature
- Standards of conduct
- Termination
- Time sheets
- Vacation
- Worker's Compensation
- Acknowledgment of receipt of employee handbook

As you can see, the subjects covered were extensive and the sections were outlined in great detail. Over the years, we had questions that touched on almost every subject in our manual. For example, disciplinary matters were handled in an equitable manner because all the appropriate steps were outlined in the policy manual. These steps had been read and acknowledged by the employee, so uncertainty was removed from the disciplinary equation.

A policy manual is a fair system and, just as important, it allows you to maintain a business-like atmosphere when dealing with employees. Emotional trauma is substantially eliminated from the professional relationship. Nevertheless, even the most professional policy manual does not totally eliminate legal confrontations.

Once, I was challenged by an ex-employee and summoned to Labor Relations court. I sent my Office Manager to represent our clinic. The case was quickly dismissed after my office manager provided the court with relevant sections out of our manual addressing the disputed issues. He also produced the form signed by the ex- employee indicating that she had read and understood the manual, The judge ruled in our favor. An unfavorable ruling would have cost us a substantial amount in back and vacation pay. That favorable decision, all by itself, paid the cost of our manual, including its updates.

Evaluating Personnel Management has an obligation to inform its employees regarding their performance. It's a no-brainer to sit at an evaluation and

> *The world is filled with willing people; some willing to work, the rest willing to let them.*
> —Robert Frost

praise your employee, especially if it is warranted. However, in the uncomfortable situation of poor performance, there must be a constructive discussion regarding the correction of the situation. A performance evaluation should be an opportunity to explain why an employee's work makes a difference, whether excellent or poor. Your staff should understand the "ripple effect" that their work has. When your staff understands how their work affects the rest of your office operations, they will give more thought to their work product.

Many managers find performance evaluations uncomfortable, especially if the employee has been below expectations. The "non-praise" evaluations require much more thought and should be liberally sprinkled with diplomacy. The employee whom you like the least should be the recipient of your highest diplomatic efforts. Following that path will better balance your evaluation interviews. I'm an advocate of a policy which separates performance evaluations from pay increases. The two should be at distinctly different times. In this way, the impact of a performance evaluation is stronger, whether it is good or bad. From the employee's standpoint, the evaluation is not tied to a pay increase.

For example, what if you have a great employee but low cash flow? When the review and raises are tied together, it is normal for an employee to wait for the "punch line" the raise at the end of the review. Separate the two and the employee will focus on your evaluation.

*Blessed is the influence of one
true, loving human soul on another.*

–George Eliot

21

Marketing

I'm A Doctor, Not A Salesman!

Chiropractic marketing is the total of the activities involved in getting your services to patients.

This includes advertising and selling.

In Webster's, "to sell" means "to persuade or influence to a course of action or to the acceptance of something." Another definition might be, "to get those who would benefit most from our chiropractic services to utilize the offered services." Isn't that what we try to accomplish when we discuss chiropractic with others?

The majority of us agree that chiropractic is not something that should be hidden away in a cave to be utilized only by an elite few. Certainly, you'll agree that sharing the life-enhancing benefits of chiropractic care with others is a service to humanity.

As a doctor of chiropractic, you are in the service business. Is it not then incumbent upon you to reach out to your fellow man and persuade or influence them to a course of action that will lead them to accept our chiropractic work as their life-enhancing benefit?

That sure sounds like selling to me!

Selling something does not have to mean getting in someone's face to push yourself and your ideas until they scream for mercy. My brother was a salesman for high-powered IBM for twenty-five years. He never got in anyone's face to sell his products. He relied on his excellent knowledge of IBM products to educate his customers, who then made informed decisions to buy IBM.

Chiropractic is an honest product. Selling chiropractic services means getting your potential patients to seriously consider what you are offering by selling your validity before you sell your services. Although I am naturally an aggressive person, especially when I believe in something, I recognized that selling my chiropractic services could be accomplished in a considerate, gentle manner. I learned early that this method of presenting chiropractic is also less stressful and more enjoyable.

My transition from the world of business to the world of chiropractic made it a natural for my planning to include selling and promoting this wonderful service to our community. Some of my colleagues looked shocked when I told them of my plans. "We're not salesmen," they would tell me, "we are doctors!"

I said, "It was my understanding that 'doctor,' in Latin, means teacher. What better subject to teach than the benefits of chiropractic? First, however, the teacher must be trusted."

The unacceptable alternative is to keep this remarkable service a secret. That was not why I established a practice in my community.

My mission was to better the health of the community in which I lived. One of my goals was to influence the community to accept chiropractic even more than they had in the past. To do this, my practice had to reach out to positively influence as much of the community as possible. Sales and promotion were the best first steps I could think of that would lead us to the accomplishment of my mission.

In order to properly build a practice, I had to sell my product. In any sales situation, establishing the credibility of the seller is a primary goal. Selling a service is more easily accomplished when the buyer believes in the person doing the selling.

I worked at showing to potential patients that I was an ethical practitioner knowledgeable about his product. When that was established, it was much easier to communicate with others on the values inherent in chiropractic care.

I was very careful to promise only what I could produce, making certain that my staff and I made only statements that could be backed up with results. This applied even to how long a patient would wait in the reception area. We never said that a patient would be able to, "get rid of (whatever) in a certain number of visits. We did, however, tell a new patient if results were not apparent within (an appropriate number of visits), we would sit down together and re-evaluate their case. If the results of that re-evaluation so indicated, I would recommend either another chiropractor or a medical specialist.

If a program or procedure is presented to a patient with a time-line, they know where they stand. Our promises to the new patient extended even to office procedures. Our policy was that the wait in the reception area would be minimal. It was therefore minimal. Appointments, the time spent waiting for treatment, the treatment program itself, all had known end points.

No con jobs were offered, nor any pie-in-the-sky promises. Honesty was our primary consideration. Any other efforts in the marketing area was secondary to this basic concept.

Marketing, Sales, Outreach, Whatever!

What's in a name? That which we call a rose by any other name would smell as sweet.
—William Shakespeare

Unless you are a hermit, you sell something. If you don't like the word sales just substitute, education, promotion, or whatever makes you feel comfortable. Influencing the consuming public regarding the health benefits of chiropractic is honorable as long as the methods are honest and ethical.

With that said, let's move forward to talk about" Whatever."

One of the first things you have to establish in your business is what your business is all about. What are you supposed to be doing? Though this seems very basic, you'd be surprised at the number of people who forget the reason their business is in existence.

We are in the business of chiropractic, with all that "business" and "chiropractic" mean to us. You already have an understanding of what chiropractic service means to you, otherwise your practice would have collapsed long before you started reading this book. Your business means having a *service* that can be honestly sold, at a profit, to the consuming public.

Marketing a Service

Chiropractors market a service, not a product. You can't see, touch, or feel a service, which is abstract, elusive, and intangible. More than that, chiropractors offer a personal service. When consumers buy chiropractic, they do it with uncertainty, discomfort, and sometimes distrust. The fact that their health is involved and that there are no guarantees only accentuate the customers' lack of assurance.

If you haven't already discovered it, you will soon learn that marketing a service like chiropractic is very different from marketing a product. As much as anything, you are marketing an intangible promise. Your clients will gauge your service by how well you keep that implied promise.

At the same time, new clients often come to you with negative expectations—all the intangible reasons they can give for saying no. They're afraid of *pain* ("I'm afraid it will hurt," or "I'm in too much pain to see you right now"). They're afraid of *commitment* ("Chiropractors make you come back forever"). They're afraid of the *cost* ("I can't afford you right now—or ever"). They're afraid of the *time* commitment ("I'm too busy with school, work, church, the garden, etc., and I just don't have time to see you")

Good marketing means being able to respond to these intangibles. If the client is afraid of pain, you can always tell them that your first order of business will be to reduce their discomfort. Go into as much detail as the patient needs to feel that pain will not be an issue.

Is the patient wary of commitment? You can reassure the patient that they will be in ultimate control of the commitment and allow them to control their future appointments after they agree to the minimum number of visits needed to address their problem. In reality, the patient is always in control of the appointment schedule, but this simple reassurance is all many patients need to feel comfortable making even a minimum commitment.

Is the patient concerned about the cost? Do something to ease the patient into the office. Perhaps you make allowances for the first visit or agree to a package discount if the patient agrees to a set number of appointments. Just make sure you aren't lowering your prices below your break even point!

Perhaps the patient is concerned about the time commitment. Show the patient you are willing to work with them by examining your schedule to find those times when you can get the patient in and out of the office with a minimum of delay. Or offer them a walk-in schedule so they can come in at their convenience even if it means an occasional wait.

Your success in marketing your service will be directly proportional to your success in marketing yourself. Show your empathy, your professionalism, and your dedication. Accommodate your patients' needs. You'll win a loyal customer.

Your Position in the Community

Developing a position means increasing your visibility in the eyes of others. Your position is a reflection of how you and your practice are perceived in the community. There is always a difference between the position you want to occupy and the position you do occupy. As closely as you can, you want to make the position you occupy resemble the position you want to occupy.

There are a number of things you can do. The first is to figure out what you want to be in the eyes of your patients and your community. You are not going to be a success by chance. The health-care industry can be very competitive. To establish *your* services in the market, you need to take some time to position your practice so that the community thinks of you first. A good position means that your patients trust your judgments, you community pays more attention to you, and your standing among local businesses goes up

In *Positioning,* Al Ries and Jack Trout list four guidelines for establishing a position in a market:

- You must position youself in your prospect's mind
- Your position should be singular in that it has one simple message
- Your position must set you apart from your competitors
- You must sacrifice, by focusing on one thing; you cannot be all things to all people

There is plenty of room for you to stake out your own unique position. Techniques aside, all chiropractors have different personalities and deliver their services differently. Use the following steps to find your own special place in the community:

Step 1: Determine the best DCs in your area. Why are they "the best"? Emulate what they do best. If you can provide services that are equally adept, do it! You'll immediately raise the perception of your practice as equal to the best.

Step 2: Listen to every person who is or might become a patient. Do this when you talk to patients in your office and do it some more when you talk to groups in the community or converse with friends, relatives, staff, and people on the street. Make a list of all the likes and dislikes people share with you. This list is worth is weight in gold. It tells you what your patients and potential patients want and what they don't think they are getting yet.

Step 3: Analyze the information you get. Useful information should jump off the page at you. Do patients want to get in and out of the chiropractic office quickly or avoid waiting a long time? Make note of it. Do potential customers demand convenient parking? Make note of it. Pay attention to the negatives, as well. Do patients believe that the only reason chiropractors take X-rays is to pad their wallets? Do they resent the time it takes to hear reports of findings? Pay attention to that, too.

Step 4: Act On Your New Information. Your position will be strengthened if your community believes you respond to their needs. If patients don't want to wait, figure out how you can develop the reputation of being the fastest chiropractor in town. If they don't understand why X-rays are needed, see if you can become the chiropractor who explains things in everyday English. If patients want parking, make sure parking and access are not problems.

Your position stakes out your claim to provide a unique service, one that distinguishes you from the other practitioners in your community. Now let the community know about your service. There are as many ways to do this are there are activities to participate in. You can advertise, which is the subject of the next chapter. Can you write? Do a periodic column for your local paper. Or hire someone to do the writing for you. Do you speak well? Make a list of local service clubs and offer a twenty-minute, informative talk on chiropractic. Do you play golf or tennis? Make friends on the local courses and courts. Teach a course at the local adult school. Offer to host your own radio show on a local station. Volunteer to be an authority-on-call for the local news media. Only your imagination limits your options.

Determining the Market for Your Services

We know our basic product is chiropractic service (For this discussion we'll set aside supplements, appliances, and so on). The next step will be to determine whom you want to reach as potential patients. Since you have already been in practice for a while, you should have an idea of your patient market. Look at your patient market a little closer and ask several questions.

Have you identified and explored the entire boundary of your patient market?

Most practice consultants agree that the basic marketing area of most practices encompass a three to five mile radius around your clinic. If you move your clinic, try to stay within that range.

There are exceptions to this rule. Many chiropractors have patients who travel long distances for treatments. Unless you have a practice that falls into that "very special" category, the majority of your patients will generally come from within that three to five mile area.

Have you communicated with your patient's family decision maker?

Be certain that your marketing efforts have been dealing with the person who makes the treatment decisions. When I examined this issue, I discovered the woman in the family made many of those decisions. The data gathered also indicated that women are more likely to take those extra steps necessary to take care of themselves more than the men. (Let's leave the reasons up to social anthropologists).

The theory was verified when our patient gender mix was checked in our office. The ratios were 2.5:1 females to males even though both males and females seemed to be equally busy with their family and work schedules.

Have you identified specialized marketing potentials within your current practice?

Seriously consider surveying the possibilities of marketing to the special interest groups represented by your current patients. This often involves their spare time activities. Sometimes their special interests will be their occupations.

When I was in active practice, I spent one weekend a month racing somewhere on the West Coast. I was involved with the amateur racing community, which, like other similar groups, was close-knit. Drivers and their crews traveled the same circuits. Their families usually traveled with them.

I knew, from personal experience, the physical and emotional stresses and the types of injuries race car drivers experienced. I also knew what advice a driver would or would not accept. Further, I was aware it was common practice for the wives and crew chiefs to try to keep their drivers as healthy as possible for two important reasons: they were personally concerned about his health, and a healthy driver has an edge over his competition.

I decided to put "Delman Chiropractic" on our race car and trailer. After a short time, I was approached at the track by some drivers and their crews inquiring about chiropractic treatment and how it might be applicable to their particular situations. I started bringing a portable table to the track setting it up next to our race car with a sign stating "Courtesy chiropractic treatment to drivers and crew." Between my races, I performed palliative work for the racers.

Increasingly, I saw drivers and those involved with racing coming to our clinic for non-courtesy treatment programs. By knowing their special lifestyles, I would tailor their treatments accordingly.

Be aware when you and your patients have strong common interests, "bench racing" with your buddies can put you far behind your schedule! To better control our appointment schedule, several of the more talkative drivers had to be scheduled at the end of the day. This prevented rioting by my impatient patients in the reception area while I yakked with my friends.

My advertising expanded to include sponsoring race vehicles in other venues, further developing that specialized market. Utilizing unique experiences, I had found a niche and was having fun in the process.

Have you found similar providers who would consider networking?

When I opened in my home town, I decided to visit other local chiropractors. I knew there was strength in networking, especially for those in solo practice. I also knew that when I ran into the inevitable "treatment stumper," it would be reassuring and helpful to be able to call a colleague to discuss that problem.

Was I was surprised at the various receptions I received! While most doctors were friendly, several were absolutely paranoiac. One doctor actually ordered me out of his office, shouting as I left, "I'm not going to share information with my competition!" What the poor man didn't understand was that professionals compete against their own goals and objectives, not against each other! You and I have the capability of doing whatever we want with our practices. It would be irrational to think that we are able to substantially influence the success or failure of another professional.

Later that week, I visited a chiropractor in another part of town. He was very helpful with local vendor information. While we were having a pleasant chat, his phone rang. It was the same chiropractor who ordered me out of his office. The chiropractor was calling, to warn the doctor I was visiting that, "Another chiropractor had moved into our town." My new friend laughed and told him, "Not to panic, He's here visiting." It was a short phone call.

There are many reasons to visit the local, established chiropractors. My reasons for visiting were simple. I wanted someone to call if I had questions involving my new practice, I needed information on local vendors and supply houses. I wanted to make certain my office was up to local standards. Finally, I wanted to see if someone would be available to cover my patients when I was out of town.

Despite my bad experience with the one doctor, I strongly recommend that you visit your local colleagues. You'll end up with mutually beneficial alliances that can last a lifetime. There were two of us in our home town who ended up using each other as a resource whenever the opportunity arose. Since he utilized a totally different technique, his office was also a good referral source when we had patients who were not responding to our treatments. We knew each other's areas of knowledge, we were honest with each other in our responses, and we utilized our resources for our mutual benefit the entire time we were in practice. We continue to be friends even though we're a continent apart.

Have you made yourself aware of economic, political and geographical trends in your market?

As part of your plan for long term growth, your patient market must be strong and stable. Your market should be capable of growth equal to your practice potential. As a businessman, it is important that you stay abreast of your market's economic and political trends.

The best way to determine a community's direction is to be involved in its activities. Patronize local stores and establishments and make an effort to meet their owners and managers. By being involved in community activities, you'll be able to meet the people who manage your local government. You will obtain insight to your community's economic direction. Knowledge of the ebb and flow of your community strengths also will provide you with indicators pointing to new areas of opportunity both for yourself and your practice plus information on the direction of your community's growth.

Some of these indicators are:

- Businesses moving into or out of town
- Does your community crime rate match up with other communities?
- Is the median age of your community's population changing?
- Local laws being considered that might hinder the future growth of your practice?
- How strong are the local Chamber of Commerce and the local government? Is their orientation well-balanced between the large and small business of your community? Have they been successful at bringing new business into your community?

You're looking for answers that reflect a vibrant, growing community. Determine if it promises to provide your practice with potential for parallel growth.

*The product that will not sell without advertising will
not sell profitably with advertising.*

–Albert Lasker

22

Advertising

To Advertise Or Not, That's The Question

Advertising, within the context of your marketing plan, is acceptable as long as the return on your investment is reasonable. The health care market's profit centers have been shrinking. Therefore, advertising costs have to shrink, especially when compared to the more profitable 1980s. Advertising has to be more targeted and precise. A clinic owner no longer has the option to spread advertising indiscriminately across the various media.

During our two years of traveling, I asked chiropractors how much they spent on marketing. Their answers ran the spectrum from "None" to "Substantial." Most did not have defined budgets, however, and many spent according to whim rather than plan. In the current, lower profit market, however, a plan is necessary.

Most small business owners spend about four percent of their revenues on advertising. According to business consultants, the percentage should be around ten percent. That should be divided between standard advertising and special creative programs. I have spent as much as fourteen or fifteen percent and as little as six percent. I was guided by the results rather than the salesmanship of an advertising representative.

The best advertising continues to be word of mouth. Referral advertising is definitely the most effective and least costly of all marketing programs. This type of advertising is called "Internal Marketing." Every practice management book I have read devotes many words toward developing effective internal marketing systems. Perhaps this is oversimplification; however, our internal marketing consisted of satisfying our patients, educating them on what they received then asking for referrals so they can help others, as they were helped. Most people have trouble asking people for something and chiropractors are no exception. There is no magic formula, if your patient is happy with your service, to ask them to refer. It's not a favor. It's an obligation! Just do it!

Wait for the time when your patient tells you how great you are. That's the time to request them to refer a friend or neighbor who needs your services. After getting over your surprise at the ease of asking, your reluctance disappears and your internal marketing program begins.

Successful Advertising Strategies

The business that considers itself immune to the necessity for advertising sooner or later finds itself immune to business.
—Derby Brown

"I'm building a referral only practice No advertising!" Well, if that's your uncompromising position on advertising, you might want to skip this section. Before you leave, though, here's something to consider. Operating your practice without advertising is like winking at a girl in the dark. You know what you're doing, but does anyone else?

Advertising your practice is not just placing an ad in the Yellow pages (lousy cost-benefit ratio) or a full page ad in your local newspaper (insanity). The key to effective advertising is consistency.

We know doctors who do no advertising. Others advertise until their wallets implode! Then there are those who are all shades of gray, in between. The whole purpose of advertising is to consistently get the "word" to your market, informing them that the service you are offering is worthy of their consideration and consumption. It usually takes ten or more ad exposures to make an impression, so don't expect immediate results.

Which of the many methods of advertising you utilize is a very personal choice.

When I first started in practice, I decided to strongly advertise my services to the community. As my practice became more well-known, I slowly decreased the amount of advertising and changed to tighter venues. I reduced our newspaper advertising, for example, and placed more emphasis on theater and cable advertising. By placing different ads in each medium, I was able to track their effectiveness. For me, the most cost-effective was cable advertising, since the majority of my marketing area was serviced by local cable.

Theater advertising was the second most effective because it advertised to a captive audience during intermission. Median strip sponsorship (see below) was next with newspaper advertising last. I used newspaper ads for several years with relatively small but consistent placements. Eventually, I stopped newspaper advertising completely, with no discernable decrease in community exposure.

It was never in our plans to totally stop advertising. It always remained in our budget.

Advertising Lessons We Have Learned

Advertising is 85% confusion and 15% commission.
—Fred Allen

We discovered that it is insane to place full page newspaper ads. It is more effective and economical to run a series of smaller ads. Again, the key to effective advertising is consistency! A big splash ad impacts only for a short period of time. A consistent advertising program saturates your intended market. Plus, a consistent ad program interfaces better with the rest of your promotional efforts. We followed the same line of thinking when we planned our cable advertising schedules.

When you purchase cable advertising on a yearly contract, benefits can be negotiated into your package. These additional perks will dramatically enhance the overall impact of your cable advertising program.

Some of the benefits we received were:

- The cable company used our ads more than those of their by-the-month advertisers. It often used our ads to fill "dead" spaces in its time slots, all at no additional charges.
- Filming new spots or changes of our existing spots were done at no cost.
- The cable company gave us the VIP customer treatment, accommodating us when we needed a crew to film one of our community events. Later, they would run those event spots more than the usual public service announcements (PSA). Many times I would be chosen to be in the event film, since I knew the cameraman and producer. All of those public service announcements were aired much closer to prime time than usual pre-dawn PSA times.

I gave the cable company permission for their sales personnel to use my ads as examples during their presentations to prospective clients. This gave us added exposure to the rest of the business community. Of course, since the sales people said we were successful because we were using cable advertising, our local business validity increased.

In no special order, here are a few of the successful concepts that guided our advertising programs:

- Determine what makes you unique as a chiropractor. What do you have to offer that will make you stand apart from the other practitioners who are going after the same market?

• Carefully craft a headline to your ad that will draw the reader into the rest of it.

• Write ad copy that will get your own unique message to your prospective patient. Writing the copy is not complicated as long as you keep four elements in mind: use a headline to grab the reader's attention; use a picture or illustration to emphasize your text; write simple ad copy that focuses on one thought; include your address and contact information.

Be careful not to write ad copy to impress your colleagues. Remember, the potential patient does not understand and will not be impressed by all your degrees and certifications. Your advertising will be more effective if you explain the unique skills you possess and how they will benefit the reader of your advertising.

• Use white space to complement the look of your printed ads. You have only a few seconds to get the attention of your reader. How many advertisements have you seen that are so full of information you only glance at them and then move on to another ad? If the reader is overwhelmed by the amount of text in your ad, then he will quickly move on to another area.

White space emphasizes the copy. An ad is not the place to educate a prospective patient. Get them to investigate your unique services. Once you get that person into your office, your exceptional staff and exceptional service will make him a valued patient.

• Don't use tacky gimmicks and giveaways. They demean our profession and cause difficulties later. If you advertise free x-rays or give away some inducement to get patients into your office, unless you are absolutely able to separate the free services from those charged, be prepared to give away freebies for a very long time.

• The courtesy services we provided at the race track were totally different from those provided in our office. We performed mostly palliative work with minimal adjusting. We advised track patients to follow up with their chiropractor. If they had none, we gave them our business card.

• A serious patient will not be enticed by gimmicks. The only no-fee service we offered in our office was our consultation. We were careful not to appear as if we were doing "bait & switch." After the consultation, if they wanted to start our recommended program, we'd schedule them for a later time. It might even be as soon as later on the same day. but never immediately! There had to be a definite separation between consultation and treatment.

We felt it was important to clearly differentiate between the a free consultation and any fee-based services.

- Stay away from strictly institutional-type advertising, the kind of ad that basically just informs the reader that you exist. An example of this type of ad might look like this:

BOREDOM CHIROPRACTIC CLINIC

1460 Rotator Road
Mytown, FL
(444) 444-4444

We've been practicing
Chiropractic a long time!

There are no benefits or demands for action in these ads. The ads might even look nice and clean. However unless your clinic's name is "Coca Cola," there's no advantage for you to run institutional-type of advertising. Effective ads start with a "grabber" headline and have inducements in them. Your advertising should contain your location, what you do, a command to take action, and, most important, a benefit to the person reading your advertisement. An ad containing those elements is below.

It's Time To Stop Hurting!

[Picture or illustration showing someone in pain]

I've been helping your neighbors for five years.
Why not you?
The only way to find out is to call me today at (123) 456-7890 to discuss your pain.

Go ahead! Pick up the phone! All you can lose is your pain!

Ivan Delman, D.C.
1465 Hotshot Highway
Happytown, TN
(Across from Soggy Oaks Mall)

Call today for your free consultation
(123) 456-7890

It only took a few minutes to put this ad together. If you write, re-write, polish, and re-polish it, you'll produce an ad that fits your practice like a comfortable glove.

No one is better able to write the words for your ad than yourself. You know your principles, your limits, and your heart. Ad arrangement, layouts, and so on, can be delegated to media specialists. However, you should have final say, because you know how far you can go and still feel comfortable. Don't be talked into anything that makes you uneasy!

The purpose of an ad is to invite a prospective patient into your clinic so you can show him or her the possibilities of chiropractic care. Make no guarantees and tell the truth.

A Secret Weapon: Your Business Card

Some drink from the fountain of knowledge. Some only gargle.
—Proverb

Business cards have power. They're "Instant Advertising" every time you hand one out. Ask yourself, "How effective is my business card? Where does it go when I hand it out?"

When I see a business card, it usually looks the same as thousands of other business cards. I throw away about ninety percent of them on the same day! Why is that? Because most cards are not special! I first heard this concept at a Jim Parker seminar. Jim's acronym still rings true today, "W.O.C .Whip Out Card at every opportunity and make your card special to the recipient."

One way to make that card special is to offer a benefit for your prospective patient right on your card. You'll greatly increase chances to sell something if you give something first. Having a strong sales tool like the word free! on your card makes it special. When you hand out a card, write on the back, *Gary, please present this card at my office for your FREE consultation. Offer expires in 30 days. Looking forward to seeing you, Dr. D. June 28, __.*

Several important sales points were covered within this short, handwritten message:

- I wrote it by hand in front of the recipient.
- I called the recipient by his first name.
- I signed it with my nickname rather than formal title and dated it.
- I offered a free consultation, which added value to the card *and added an expiration date.*

For efficiency, all of the above can also be pre-printed on the back of your card, since you probably have a standing-free consultation policy.

To help advertise my presence, I used to leave my cards in phone booths, on community bulletin boards, and in gas stations. Whenever I was in our library, I placed business cards in as many health-oriented books as possible. In restaurants, my server always got his or her tip with a note written on the back of my card expressing my thanks for their excellent service.

Once you start thinking creatively about using your business card, the possibilities are extensive. So, take a good look at your business card. It's your secret weapon!

Writing Your Own Advertising Copy

All I know is what I see in the papers.
—Will Rogers

If you're going to write your own ad copy or, if you want to properly monitor someone who is writing your copy, here are some useful guidelines:

- Remember, the reason you are writing this ad is to sell (inform, teach) the reader on your chiropractic services.
- Do not make incredible statements. Even if true, it'll make you look unbelievably self-serving.
- Start with a grabber then progress systematically through your ad, ending with a contact number. A grabber is some line of type that is designed to "grab" a passing reader. Here are some examples of what we used. You write whatever fits your philosophy and standards:

   Tired Of Pain?
   Want Health, Naturally?
   How Long Since You've Felt Good?
   Tired Of Drugs?
   Gentle Treatment

- Keep your words to a minimum. Otherwise, your message becomes a heap of words. What is your message? Make sure it satisfies these four parameters:

   Who you are
   What you provide
   When can you provide it
   Where you provide it.

- Stick to a singular theme. If you try to be a doctor for all reasons, it becomes hard for the reader to associate with all those multiple themes.
- Be professional! In Chiropractic advertising, humor is not usually warranted (although it can be tempting!). Your ad must reflect you without embarrassing your practice or your profession. Don't advertise prices. If you have reasonable first visit fees or offer family plans, sharing that information is best handled after the patient contacts your office.
- Use a lot of white space. Let the reader quickly find your message instead of having to dig it out from a landfill of verbiage.

• Make the benefits stand out in your ad. Here are some examples of a benefit:

> *regain your health*
> *low cost treatment programs*
> *don't wait unnecessarily for treatment*
> *in most cases, covered by insurance*
> *70 years experience*
> *emergency service.*

Benefits and a "grabber" line look similar, but they are not. The "grabber" line is designed to be quickly spotted and carries more emotion whereas the benefit takes a little longer to absorb.

For the print media, I designed ads with more white space than text. It had the essentials, a professional picture, and not much more. They were small and ran consistently.

• Above all, be truthful! From a legal standpoint, you will get nailed if you promise what you cannot deliver. From an ethical standpoint, it is imperative for your community credibility and your own self-worth to be honest. Be honest not only about the service, which is honest in itself, but the offers ("Emergency availability," "we cure toad's warts," etc.) Only offer what you are able and willing to provide! Consider "emergency availability." This is included in just about everyone's advertising. However, just try to get some of those doctors on a weekend! If you advertise you have emergency service, be prepared to answer your pager. Yes, there are times when the call is not really an emergency. They can be handled. We all have had the "emergency" patient who never returned and stiffed you on payment, besides. But, there will be more times when your emergency care has been appreciated by the caller. In fact, whenever there is an emergency, you have the opportunity to build strong patient loyalties just by opening your office to handle that emergency. As long as you tell parents when you're available, they'll understand.

We left once every month for three days of racing. Our patients knew that, and we even changed the recording on our answering machine to indicate our activity that weekend. My patients made appointments either before or after the race weekend. I don't believe our practice suffered from our not being available during a race weekend. I also believe that patients are reluctant to change doctors unless that patient is seriously unhappy with his service.

The importance of being available for emergency service was emphasized during our first few years of practice. I received an emergency call from a local insurance salesman who, prior to that call, had been an infrequent patient. He usually determined his own treatment protocol. One Sunday he placed an emergency call saying he had fallen while trying to jump over a fence. He was in a world of hurt, quite literally! I told him to meet me at the clinic in 30 minutes. After examining him, I did some palliative work and told him to return the next day to continue treatment. After a few visits, all ended well and he was a happy patient. More than that, he became compliant to our recommendations. Lastly, he told everyone he met about our excellent service. He continued to refer patients for at least,10 years.

How much was that hour on Sunday worth?

Other Types of Advertising

We advertised in other media beside the newspapers. When we stopped newspaper advertising, we exclusively used these three following venues:

Cable TV: We used a different concept here, since we could get the viewer to better visualize our service. I obtained ready-made chiropractic commercials from a quality VHS producer of chiropractic commercials. There were sections of the tape (called donuts) designed for us to insert personalized spots regarding our clinic. In exchange for a year's contract with the cable company, the cable company brought their equipment to our office where we made the inserts. I chose the inserts we'd utilize. I obtained, then studied, the demographics of each cable channel. Our selection of channels to run our commercials was based upon our clinic's profiles. The commercials were run on a rotational basis to keep them fresh. As I pointed out earlier, since we contracted for a year, the cable company ran those commercials, at no cost, as fill-ins on other channels during late and other non prime-time hours. This saturated most of the available channels for a reasonable cost.

In our town, cable TV advertising enjoyed an excellent market due to poor regular antenna reception. The cable advantage placed us at least on a par with network advertisers. Local cable advertising is substantially less expensive than most other TV media.

Theater advertising: This was another effective venue to increase our exposure to the community. Theater advertising is a slide program produced, at no charge, by a theater advertising agency. The slides are shown during intermissions between movies. Advertiser's slides are interfaced with movie quiz slides and other advertising. The slide is designed to be read in 3 seconds. The mix of advertising and informational slides kept the attention of the audience. I was able to directly connect obtaining new patients to my theater advertising programs.

City median strips: Sponsoring certain sections of city landscaping is a good example of a consistent advertising program. Some cities offer business owners opportunities to sponsor the maintenance of selected city-owned properties. In exchange for a low monthly fee, the city will erect a visible sign indicating the maintenance of that city property was sponsored by a specific business. Those signs not only advertised our business, but implied we were civic-minded as well.

We picked high-flow areas on streets near our clinic. Getting the signs as close to your clinic as possible adds to the effectiveness of other signs on or near your clinic.

A Final Advertising Thought

The safest way to double your money is to fold it over once and put it in your pocket.
—Kin Hubbard

Many practice management consultants advise you to watch the *Return On Investment* (ROI) in your expenditures, especially when you are putting out bottom line dollars, such as advertising. If you add up your advertising dollars and divide it by the number of new patients you obtain for those dollars, the result tells you what it cost to acquire new patients. The idea is to have a "reasonable" return on your advertising investment per patient.

ROI is a valid concept. However, I never seemed to get around to living by that figure. I tried several methods to evaluate our advertising expenditures, finally settling on connecting our advertising budget to a percentage of our gross income.

As our gross income increased, so did our advertising/marketing budget. We wasted many dollars and churned through numerous advertising programs before ending up with a percentage (six to ten percent) that seemed to work well for our type of practice. Marketing is an imperfect science with advertising falling under that umbrella.

Advertising can familiarize potential patients with your offered services. It does not guarantee to bring in new patients just because your text is awe-inspiring, your credentials heroic, or your picture pretty. It will not make the sale. It does, however, help bring patients to your practice. Your advertising outreach has to be complemented and balanced by other activities such as community involvement, special clinic programs, and so on. The combination of all those activities makes getting out the "word" effective.

All the world's a stage,
And all the men are merely players.
They have their exits and their entrances,
And one man in his time plays many parts.
—William Shakespeare

23

On Looking As You Wish To Be

As your office grows, you should start thinking about divesting yourself of extra chores you have been handling. These should be delegated to a responsible staff member or sub-contacted to an outside provider.

When we were in our first office, we personally cleaned the entire office at the end of each work day On our off days, we mowed the lawn and kept the landscaping looking presentable. We also heard a few comments from patients about the "doctor doing his own lawn?"

At one of his seminars, Jim Parker said, "Act and look like a successful doctor at all times you are in the public eye. This includes what you wear and what you drive."

That statement was driven home one day while I was standing outside my office. I had just installed a new sign and was admiring it while resting from mowing the lawn. A passing pedestrian saw me standing looking up at the sign. He stopped and asked me what I thought about, "That new doctor in there" and "Did he do a good job" and "Would I go back to him?"

Of course, I went on enthusiastically telling this person how great the doctor was and how happy all of his patients were with the results of his treatments.

That person eventually presented as a patient and we both had a pretty good laugh. It did remind me, however, that whenever I was around the office, I had better look like "The Doctor." Whether we like it or not, initial impressions are powerful. A patient is not going to take advice as seriously if it comes from Yoda the gardener.

Since I don't like wearing a tie, I wore loose, colored jackets. I also got rid of the Junker I had been driving and bought a cleaner, newer car. I was amazed at the difference in attitude from both new and old patients. It was subtle but it was there.

From then on, I wore what I considered appropriate attire during patient hours. I also required and paid for comfortable, colorful uniforms and name tags for our staff. I hired someone to cut the lawn, someone to clean the office, and someone to keep the car I was driving repaired and clean.

I knew my local image improved. Whether that made a major contribution to the success of my practice, I can't definitively say. However, Jim's advice helped me remember what part I was playing during that stage of my life.

"All of us belong to a greater whole, and whether you call it society or civilization or country, it has a deep and profound impact on our lives. Some seek to escape it. Some to embrace it. All of us, though, should seek to understand it"

–anon

24

Lessons Others Have Taught Me

I've learned a number of lessons from my mentors and from the horrendous mistakes I have made. I sincerely hope that sharing them with you will save you from having to salvage the wreckage of no-win decisions:

Choices If your life stinks that's because you've made the decision to pick up a dead fish. You didn't have to pick up that fish. It was your choice.

We all know people who have a history of failure, people who consistently make poor business decisions and who fail much too often. When you discuss the reasons for the failure, they'll tell you how someone else goofed up, took advantage of them or whatever. This type of thinking tends to destroy an endeavor right out of its starting gate.

If you choose a course of action and expect to lose, you will!

Examine why these people consistently fail. Probably, their failures result from the poor choices that they keep repeating. Their poor choices are often caused by their negative mind-set. Those poor folks expect to lose…and they fulfill their expectations. Their negative mindset will be changed only if that person decides to change it.

I once needed an office manager who could handle the details of our office operations and for several other businesses. I also needed someone to supervise the employees of those ventures. My friend Mark was looking for a job and had the skills I was looking for. When I first talked to him, he held a management job with an international company. However, he repeatedly told me that they were not letting him do a proper job and it was a dead-end deal.

So I hired Mark. He proved to be an excellent manager, and I compensated him accordingly for his good work. We got along great, and the employees loved his style of management. After about a year, however, his old pattern reared its ugly head. He told me the job for which I hired him was, "A dead-end job…I feel stymied…etc." He resigned (amicably) to look for another job.

He went on to hold three other jobs, all with the same results and the same faulty reasoning. One day, Mark and I had a talk. He was concerned that he was approaching age 50 with no savings, no current career, and slim hopes for the future. Mark and I talked seriously about his attitude. He finally understood how he was responsible for his own luck. He accepted that he had to reprogram himself to succeed. He also recognized that he needed to understand and control his choices.

Mark finally returned to his old international company in a different management position. He had a new positive attitude. He felt his future had a brighter outlook. I wished him well and I know he'll be happier in his accomplishments.

If you find yourself in this type of situation, don't look around for someone else to blame. You're in control; only *you* can change your course of action. If you're unhappy with where you are, then take control! Start by understanding the type of decisions you are making.

Make a list of all the actions that brought you to this undesirable position. Look at each decision you have made and action you have taken and ask if they added or subtracted from your undesirable result. I'll be very surprised if you don't see a pattern of poor choices. Be aware of the decisions that did not work out and make your new decisions accordingly. Don't keep repeating the unsuccessful ones. Folly is doing the same thing that has never worked but expecting it to work this time. If that sounds simplistic, it is, but it makes right decisions much easier to make.

Promote With Class

You don't need gimmicks to be successful. Playing with flashy promotional devices is okay only if you want to have some fun. They are not, however, long-term avenues to the success you desire.

You could offer three-dollar adjustments, for example, and get lots of takers for that offer. What that will do is establish, in the minds of your patients, that your services are worth only three dollars. In the short run, you'll get new patients. In the long run you'll lose your professional value and authority.

There's nothing wrong in trying to make it easier for new or current patients to use your services. How you go about doing that is more important. Your services must remain valuable to your patient.

For example, you can give your son a car or you can make him earn it. He will appreciate and take better care of that car if he earns it, because he exchanged value for it. If you simply give him the car, he has no incentive to value it. Easy come, easy go. Giving away your services works the same way.

Things like free consultations to evaluate new patient concerns, payment plans, and reduced charges for the first visit will not decrease the value of your services in the patient's eyes. Gimmicks will. Chicken dinners, gifts, and free visits to induce new patient input are not long-term tools for success. The most important part of your business is you. A foundation of credibility, expertise, and ability to deliver what you promise is an excellent basis upon which to build a healthy practice.

Associate With Winners Associate with losers and you become "An Associate in losing." Run with the winners and you'll become a top runner. I learned this when I was racing cars. I spent time with drivers who had histories of winning. I chose a Crew Chief who had multiple championships as a driver/mechanic. He was a proven winner. His experiences, along with the lessons I learned from other drivers, was essential to the success we had in our road-racing program.

When I opened my chiropractic practice, I followed the same path. I avoided people who wasted my time by throwing up their hands and blaming everything and everyone but themselves for their lack of achievement. I associated with successful chiropractors who were confident enough in their own abilities to share with me the methods that helped achieve their success.

Ethics Do Matter It's difficult to believe in yourself or your work if you're not proud of the manner in which you conduct your business. Your work ethic must measure up to the high principles by which you guide your life.

Work with passion. When you do anything with passion, you'll lways have a better chance of succeeding. You cannot have dedi - cation or passion if you're just "putting in time" on the job. If your reason for becoming a chiropractor was just the money, you'll be unhappy and eventually burn out. If your purpose is higher, you'll ignite your dedication and passion.

Showcase Your Talent The most effective way to market the merits of chiropractic is to market your own merits. Experts call this "Relational Salesmanship." Building good relationships with those you want to deal with makes sense. Remember the saying, "Would you buy a car from that person?" The importance of the product, in the eyes of the consumer, is often secondary to the importance of the provider. If your prospective patients believe you have a good grasp of your job and your business, they will want to use your services.

There are three essential concepts that must be covered when you discuss chiropractic with potential patients. You must:

- Learn the chiropractic needs of that person
- Thoroughly understand that you are offering an intangible service
- Be able to convey the unique aspects of your services in a positive manner without downgrading similar providers.

Validate your Chiropractic message by showing your patients the assets they consider important to the success of their treatment. Your expertise, experience, dedication, and your history of treatment success will all validate you in the eyes of your patient. Once your patients believe in you, they will believe in your work.

A Synergistic Suggestion You will have a strong practice if you combine personal and business motivations. If your work involves what you strongly desire to accomplish as a doctor and goals you've set for your business, your chance of making a positive difference in your community is much greater. That's because you have now added passion to your purpose. As a chiropractor with earnest aspirations, let your work transcend your job and become a lifelong mission.

To the question of your life, you are the only answer.
To the problems of your life, you are the only solution.
—Anon

25

Making It All Work

Think back to all the practice management seminars you have attended. The presenters, with tremendous energy and occasionally great showmanship, shared mountains of terrific ways to make your practice bigger and/or better.

At the end of the seminar, you rushed out of the hotel, wildly waving your arms, ready to make major changes in your practice. By the time Monday rolled around, you were a little less enthusiastic. Perhaps later that week you tried several of the new ideas then let the follow-up slide because you were so "busy." After a few weeks, the seminar was a distant memory and your practice was about in the same place as it was before the seminar.

The seminars didn't fail, you failed the seminars.

If every page in this book were made of solid gold and the ideas on them diamonds, they all would be worthless unless you took action to implement the ideas and thoughts on these pages. You, the CEO of your own practice, must start the ball rolling. You must figure out by figuring out the steps you will take on the road to practice improvement. Then, you must put those steps to work and keep them working.

No one but you can implement the seminar information that will move your practice closer to your goals. No one but you can take the information offered on these pages and choose the parts you'll use and the goals and achievements you'll strive for. No one but you can figure out how to accomplish your goals without exhausting your finite supplies of resources like time or money.

Whenever you make changes in your practice, do it in small increments. Why? Because small changes are easier to measure and correct, if necessary. If you do mess up, it'll only set your progress back a small step.

Finding out what works   The first key to making changes toward a powerful, profitable clinic is to evaluate your current operating procedures. For example, do you:

- Emulate a dictator or a wet noodle as a manager?
- know what's going on in your office or take your staff's word for it?
- Attend seminars and make huge, procedural changes to your practice or make changes in small, results-definable increments?
- Have your employees share their reports and suggestions at your weekly meetings or allow them to sit there, eyes at half-mast, while you pontificate?
- Have a telephone protocol that prevents interruptions to the attention you pay to your patients or allow patients waiting in the other room to overhear your conversations to your stockbroker?
- Limit the amount of time patients wait in your reception area or serve them lunch as they wait for their morning appointment?
- Make service commitments to your community or ignore the community that supports your practice?
- Have effective collection procedures or operate a chiropractic philanthropy?

When you look closely at the way your practice functions and start making incremental changes, you'll notice a new smoothness to your operations. While you're making progress, your work and your personal life will begin fitting into their proper places. Even if not every change works out the way you want it to, you'll remain on the proper track as long as most of your decisions are the right ones. It is normal for some decisions not to be beneficial. It's okay to occasionally go the wrong way. Only if you continue repeating wrong decisions would it be wise to question and revamp your decision-making process.

As an example, we all know people who make decisions while on the run. They do no research and they react to situations rather then act to handle them. There are some talented people who are successful at making quick decisions, but for us "normals," success will be more likely if we stop and analyze our possible moves and their results before we decide on a particular course of action. You can use a "Ben Franklin" lists or any other comparative analysis that guides you into thinking about the consequences of your actions.

When you make decisions, give yourself the advantage by doing a little research before you step on the accelerator.

Decision-Making Made Easy

Trying to be right all the time is a very subtle way of being wrong.
—Sanford Manley

There are no warning sirens, light system, or even statistics that tell you when your decision is right or wrong. The consequences will soon inform you. Good decision-making is a learned trait that becomes even more effective when the process is coupled with the willingness to take reasonably calculated risks. Your decisions will have a higher chance of being beneficial when you follow these four steps:

Define the problem: When you start analyzing a problem or situation, look at all sides. Understand the entire picture. Otherwise, you'll end up like Joe, the impetuous bungee jumper.

Joe (who lives in San Diego) and his friend Frank were driving near Tijuana, Mexico. As they crossed over an especially tall bridge, Joe slammed on the brakes and excitedly said, "This is the perfect bridge to take a bungee jump!" He hurriedly parked the car, pulled out his bungee rope, tied it to the bridge's railing and then to his ankles. As he jumped, he happily waved to Frank.

Frank watched the rope go tight as Joe approached the ground underneath their bridge. Then, it loosened as Joe flew back up on the first bounce. As the bungee returned Joe back up toward the top of the bridge, Frank was horrified to see Joe bleeding from head wounds and he noticed Joe's shirt almost torn off his body. It took four bounces before Frank could reel in the rope and each time Joe bounced back, he looked worse.

Finally, Joe was able to climb back over the railing, whereupon he collapsed on the street. Frank said, "You look terrible!" Joe replied, "Good grief. I'll never do that again! Each time I got close to the ground, a group of crazed people under this bridge hit me on the head with sticks. By the way, what's a pinata?"

Joe failed to assess his total situation. In doing that, Joe greatly increased the risks inherent in his hurried bungee jump. The moral here is to look before you leap. When you carefully assess your situation, you'll have fewer bruises.

Make every "Plan B" you can think of: Every "Plan B" is a viable alternative to your main direction. For example, if you are having difficulty finding a suitable person for a full-time position, you might decide to add two part-timers. Many of these decisions can become obvious if you look around your practice and think of the alternatives. Work these moves out prior to the possible need. It follows from Murphy's Law that events that requires management intervention almost always occur at an inappropriate time. Having a "Plan B" that you have analyzed and pre-approved will increase the chances of its success.

Prioritize your possible solutions: At times, there are so many possible solutions to your problem that your head starts spinning like a weather vane in a hurricane. Sort everything out by listing all the possible Pro's and Con's you can imagine. Wait a day, look at the list, then pick your best solutions.

Do it and evaluate the results: You'd be surprised how many people have trouble making a decision. Many people are afraid of making mistakes. If you're a manager, you don't have that luxury. Calculate your risk and make a decision. If you make no decision, you guarantee failure.

Why You Need An Information Partner

There is no such thing as a self-made man. We are made up of thousands of others.
—George Adams

Paraphrasing the words of George Adams, to succeed, we need the shared knowledge of our more experienced colleagues.

A while back, I received an e-mail that said, "Ivan, I envy you. You must have grown up in a business-oriented environment. That's the reason you are naturally predisposed to making good business decisions while I have to struggle trying to figure out my next move. Ivan, the environment you grew up in is the reason your practice and business ventures were profitable."

The above e-mail was only partly true; my ventures in and out of business haven't always been successful or profitable. Any successful venture was the result of a higher percentage of right vs. wrong decisions.

I don't believe that people are born with the tools for success tightly clasped in their neonatal hands. Although, acknowledging the quick learners, the majority of us laboriously achieve our victories because of our positive and negative learning experiences. My own positive experiences have usually involved a teacher who shared their information and experience.

I was lucky to be born into a family with a father who was a very smart businessman. During the depression years of the late 20s my Dad began his working life by sweeping floors. Most of his education was acquired on the street or in the workplace. By the time he retired in the late 1950s, he owned many of those floors he used to clean. At 92, his attitude continues to be strong and aggressive; his mind is sharp and he continues to stay up-to-date on the world of business.

Despite his age, my father continues to observe and act from a position of constant growth, as did his forward-thinking immigrant mother. He keeps up with the times and he maintains an outlook that is emphatically not old-fashioned. To this day, Dad continues to be my information partner. One of the many things he advises is "always be willing to learn without losing your temper or self-confidence."

Because of my Dad, I have always sought out coaches to help me succeed. I've been fortunate to find erudite mentors throughout my life to help inspire me in my work and my hobbies. Coaches have helped me achieve goals in less time and with fewer resources than if I would have tried to re-invent that wheel on my own.

In Chiropractic College, I had two great mentors, fellow students Herman and Dave. Herman, who was several years older, helped me understand the basics of adjusting. Dave, who is a lot younger and smarter, showed me how to study and pass the boards. When I went into practice, I visited almost all of the chiropractors in my town. Some were so threatened that they wouldn't say much more than hello. One even shouted me out of his office. I finally found one who had been successfully operating for several years and was willing to share his experiences.

I highly recommend you find a chiropractic mentor who has become successful and is willing to share his or her experiences with you. Most self-confident people who have accomplished much in their life will not be threatened by sharing their successful methods with you. They know, as did the late Dr Jim Parker, that "a candle will not lose any light by lighting another."

Whatever our current ability levels, to keep a competitive edge and to continue improving our skills, we all need a coach. I've had business coaches, racing coaches, chiropractic coaches, and guitar coaches. Many of today's top sports and business figures employ coaches to stay competitive.

A brief browse through the Internet will introduce you to the enormous variety of coaching services that are offered. The number of coaching services available just about equals the number of squirrels dropping acorns on our driveway. At one time coaching services were limited to large companies. Now, they are tailored to the small businessperson as well.

Although specific styles may vary, one central thread runs through most coaching systems. Most coaches emphasize the importance of changing yourself internally. They all work to strengthen your vision, modify your thinking, and change your protocols. These internal changes will guide you as you start to adjust your external procedures and environment. All this is directed to help you better manage your practice and your life. You have to feed the inner man before the outer one can do a decent job.

Only Use What's Comfortable

Being able to share the experiences of successful people is only the first half of the equation. The other half is being aware of what to use and what to discard. Over the years, I have kept the advice that worked for me and discarded the rest. Unfortunately, there were times I forgot what I should have remembered. Once I neglected to take my own advice and hired a close relative. Even though this really messed up my practice, firing her was an emotional chore! Nevertheless, most of the advice that I felt comfortable enough to take became integral parts of my operating philosophy.

How do you know the advice your coach shares with you will be to your benefit? You have to know the validity of your information sources. There are, in addition, a few rules of thumb for evaluating your mentor.

Your coach must:

- Be someone who has proven to you they can be trusted.
- Understand your practice mission and goals.
- Be around for questions and not disappear into a mountain cave after offering advice.
- Encourage your efforts without making judgmental declarations (including aggravating "I-Told-You So" comments).
- Offer practical information to help you over operational speed bumps.
- Not let you off the hook if you procrastinate about implementing the suggestions you've agreed to put into effect.
- Have a history of success in the areas where you need mentoring and the ability to help you be just as successful.
- Above all, have enough self-confidence to want you and your practice to succeed.

No matter how smart or successful my coach, I only used advice that fit my personal operating principles. I've seen seminar-givers pontificate on how this item or that method would change your practice life. It was successful for the advice-giver. It may not work for the advice-taker. I've seen colleagues try to implement odd advice even when they knew it was almost alien from their own methods of practice. I was not surprised when the changes my colleagues tried to bring about failed. "If you own it, it'll work, and if you don't...."

No matter how good the information is and no matter how well it worked for your advisor, unless you can apply it enthusiastically, don't use it. On the other hand, if you can "own" that advice, it can change an ordinary practice into a daily adventure, regardless of the information or product you are attempting to pass on to another human.

Rubber Walls For Your Goals

Your goals, minus your doubts, equal your reality.
—Ralph Marston

You and your employees will progress only by small steps if your goals are set too deep within your comfort zone. Set your goals outside your comfort zone. You will embrace the natural challenge to move beyond your comfort zone to attain your goals. The end result will be much greater accomplishments. The challenge of motivating yourself is often much less than the challenge of bringing your staff up to your level of motivation.

The ingredient necessary to elevate your staff is your strong sense of motivation. Money is not the mainstay of motivation. Money is one of the rewards for good work, but once that question is settled there's more to be done. If you are a progressive manager, you will institute other systems beyond the financial in order to motivate and increase the productivity of your employees.

One way to help your employees feel more motivated is to change the quality of their work environment. It's true that work is work and that if it were always fun we'd call it a hobby. So how do you increase the quality of the job? Start by considering changing the ways your staff performs their jobs:

Most employees positively respond to self-supervision within their jobs. Review the description of just one job, such as Front Desk Receptionist. Good job descriptions provide guidance for employees, but see if the job description is overly structured. If the employee is able to handle the front-desk business, is there something else they can do to provide a new and different challenge? If so, arrange it so they can do it on their own without having to talk to you or a supervisor first.

Involve your employees in the operation of your practice. Let them participate in decisions that affect their jobs and environment. Do this openly at the weekly staff meetings you hold even if you have only a two-person office.

Don't just report back to your employees about the wonderful things you learned at the prior weekend's practice seminar. Ask if some employees might be interested in attending a C.A. training or some other business seminar with you. Start small with local events and gauge the participation. Hosting your staff at faraway seminars can put a large dent in your budget. If your staff goes just for the social aspects of the trip, you've wasted your money.

(If you ask a staff member to take a class on coding and billing, even if you do pay all the bills, it's only fair to let them take a class they want to, such as chiropractic office decoration.)

Look the unused space in your office. See if it can be converted into a lounge where your staff can take undisturbed breaks or eat lunch. If so, respect that area as theirs as long as employees follow your guidelines on how much time they spend in that area. Let your employees participate. The last time I built an office, my staff designed their own break room after I showed them the space that would be devoted to it. They put everything in it, from their own bulletin board to a small refrigerator and microwave. They kept it clean and I stayed out of it.

If you want to get your staff and your practice moving forward with the least resistance, one of the first things you must understand is the unwritten rules at play in your office. One of these rules is that failure is often equated with personal failure instead of being accepted as just a bump on the road to accomplishment. Failure can be a wall that stops you cold or merely an inconvenience. If you encourage the attitude in your office that it's merely a speed bump, you'll eliminate the unwritten rule that says, "Trying something new and not succeeding is a sign of personal failure." One way to stifle accomplishment is to make disappointment a failure instead of a pause in your forward progress.

Think "outside the box." Don't be like the group of chimps that lived at the edge of a forest near a tribal village. The tribe lit campfires at night around its periphery to keep away unwanted and dangerous animals. One curious chimp approached a fire and tried to touch it and, of course, got burned. After several tries he quit. Several other chimps tried it, with the same results. The burned chimps taught the other chimps in the group to stay away from the fire.

When the chimps that were first burned passed on, they left the other chimps knowing only not to touch fire but not knowing why. After several generations, the chimps know that fire is something to stay away from. They will continue to stay within that box until some chimp thinks outside the box and stirs the fire with a stick.

When you look for solutions, consider restrictive in-the box thinking to be a way of staying in the box. Truly creative problem solving means breaking down the confines of the box and exploring a much bigger menu of solutions.

The Importance Of You In Your Practice

To get your team to cohesively work and accomplish together, start with a challenging goal, one that is reachable but not easily. Then be sure your team understands why reaching that goal will be to their benefit. ("This practice will fail in a year if we don't do this" or "We won't be able afford raises as long as things continue this way" are good ways to begin.)

Next, help your staff see the overall operation rather than their own individual functions. They have to understand that the problems in one department affect all the others. The operation of your practice depends on the smooth operations of all.

Solicit suggestions from the entire staff. Implement as many as you can. Some will work quickly and some will take longer, but all the good suggestions will move your practice toward the next level.

To get your group to work as a team, make sure they share a team commitment. If they say, "I'll see," or "I'll give it a try," they are not promising to give it their commitment. Each staff member must promise to be responsible for their actions. This responsibility must include a plan of action with timelines and intended results.

Here's where you shine as the hitch pin that holds your practice together. As the leader, your job is performed like an enzyme; that is, you affect the team's reactions without entering into them. You offer a fine form of guidance with the intention of strengthening the commitment of your staff to accomplishing the goals of their jobs and your practice.

I'd close by wishing you "good luck." But luck has nothing to do with success. Luck comes to those who make themselves ready to be lucky. You don't make yourself ready by sitting on your dreams and waiting for them to hatch. You have to start the practice ball rolling and keep it moving. For your ideas to work, they have to be made to work. You will obtain whatever level of success you plan to achieve, but nothing will happen while you are waiting to begin.

So go out and make it happen! I'm cheering for you. I look forward to hearing about your success!

*If you are out to describe the
truth, leave elegance to the tailor.*
—Albert Einstein

26

A Short Recap

- Stasis is contrary to nature. You either grow or shrink. It's your decision!
- Think success (whatever that means to you) and you will be as you think!
- Honesty, both to yourself and others, must be an integral part of your thinking process.
- Wish is a four letter word. It is permissible, when used, to germinate your chosen direction, but you must make that wish happen. That's when you use those other four letter words, goal, plan, and work.
- Stay focused on your goals. When you lose sight of your goals, you will not know where you are or where you are going.
- Be decisive! Once you have sufficient data, go for it; make that decision! Error by omission can create as much damage as error by commission.
- Listen! You can't hear very much with your mouth wide open.
- Mobile Management is a useful tool in your office. Always be aware of how your office is operating. Observing office operations on a consistent basis will enhance that awareness.
- You are a salesman AND a businessman. Working within reality will allow you to pursue your practical and ideological goals.
- To serve, you must survive!

Until we meet at one of our seminars, I sincerely wish you success in accomplishing your goals and moving beyond them.

Victory and defeat are each of the same price
—Thomas Jefferson

Sources, Resources, And Recommended Reading

Greg Stanley's, Whitehall Seminars.

This erudite gentleman was my initial inspiration to work toward a debt-free working environment. His suggestions were also crucial to helping me raise my practice of three years to a higher level of accomplishment. I strongly recommend his seminar series. They are fact-filled sans hype.

***Effective Small Business Management*, Scarborough & Zimmerer, 1996.**

In my opinion, this is one of the best and most comprehensive textbooks on this subject. It is currently being used as the textbook for small business management college courses. There is an immense amount of detailed data covering the entire small business spectrum. I strongly recommend adding this book to your permanent library.

***Executive Decision Making*, Jones, 1957.**

This was the textbook used during my business degree studies. I thought it might be outdated, however, when I re-read it, I found the principles as pertinent now as forty years ago. Their thoughts on goals is especially well described.

***The Small Business Handbook,"* Irving Burstiner.**

This is an excellent reference book written by one of the experts in this field.

***Words That Sell*, Richard Bayan.**

This book is a type of thesaurus containing high-powered words, phrases and slogans that are applicable for anyone writing any copy that is intended to sell a product.

***Growing A Business*, Paul Hawken, 1987**

The content of this book was originally shown on a PBS business series. Mr Hawken's writing style is laid-back and filled with anecdotes both from his own successful enterprises and other well-know companies. He addressed as much business philosophy as hard business facts. I found his philosophy to be realistic and informative and written with generous amounts of good humor.

***Running A One-Person Business*, Whitmyer & Raspberry, 1994.**

This book is the first time I have seen the word, "Tradeskills" which defined is "a whole cluster of behavioral attributes that are vital to running a business." Their book covers the gamut of solo business operations. Some of the book's content is devoted to home office operations and start-up procedures; however, solid business basics are included in their discussions.

***Small Business For Dummies*, Eric Tyson.**

I have ½ dozen "Dummies" books in my library covering topics such as computers, time management and salesmanship. The "Dummies" books are written with solid facts covered by chocolate-covered humor. They make great easy-to-read reference books. This book has information which also covers business startup but later in the book they get into useable business operating information.

***Joysticks, Blinking Lights, and Thrills: How to Have Fun and Success in Your Small Business*, Joseph Sherlock.**

Don't let the long title put you off from reading the excellent case studies in this book. The author illustrates problems we all have already or will run into while managing our practices.

Sources, Resources, And Recommended Reading

***The Prentice Hall Small Business Survival Guide: A Blueprint for Success*, Richard Pteris and Michael Cross.**

There is good cost-trimming information contained in this book outlined in a logical sequence. The information contained is applicable to a chiropractic practice as well as any other small business.

Archives of the Small Business Administration.

There is a gold mine of information contained in this website. Well worth mining it!

***Bootstrapper's Success Secrets: 151 Tactics for Building Your Business on a Shoestring Budget*, Kimberly Stansell.**

The information in this book is basically covered in others, however, I recommend this book when you are looking for an extensive list of business information resources.

***Beating the Odds in Small Business*, Tom Culley.**

The straight-forward manner in which the author states his facts, coupled with excellent anecdotes is what drew me to this book. If you have been in practice for more than several years, this may be too basic for you.

"*Winning The Entrepreneur's Game*, David E, Rye.

The manner in which this author delineates the attributes of an entrepreneur parallels that of a solo practitioner. It doesn't mean you'll fail if you don't "make the list." It helps point out areas that need a higher degree of attention in order for you to be successful.

Sterling Management seminars.

I credit their seminar on statistical management to my better understanding of the significance of "The numbers."

***Business Rescue*, Al Rosen.**

This author has good information regarding the methodology of turning around a business that is in decline. It is mainly pointed toward a larger business than a solo practitioner, however, some of the principles are interesting and thought-provoking.

***Small Business Survival Guide*, Robert E. Fleury.**

Excellent basic business information.

How to Run a Small Business, J.K. Lasser Institute.

This book is more related to an encyclopedia than textbook. This is not be taken as a negative comment. If you are adding reference books to your business library, this fits the bill. I especially like the way personnel management is delineated for the initiated.

Growing Your Own Business, Gregory Kishel.

The attraction in this book is the manner the author explains the transition of a business from the startup phase up to the next level. He also nicely covers taxes and the controlling factors involving personnel management.

Common Sense Management (Help for the Small Business), Milt Thomas.

This book presents realistic solutions to the various problems the owner of a small business would face. The anecdotes are interesting, humorous and pertinent.

Business of Chiropractic Publications

1227 Cedar Hill Road
Dandridge, TN 37725
(253) 484-3475 (fax)
www.businessofchiropractic.com

Dear Reader,

Many professionals like yourself have found the ideas and suggestions in this book to be worth far more than the purchase price. I hope you, too, have found *The Business of Chiropractic* to be both informative and helpful. Please let me know if you have any comments about this book or suggestions for future editions!

You can keep up with our latest informative articles on how to be a successful manager of your practice by visiting our web site, www.businessofchiropractic.com.

While you are there, please subscribe to our free newsletter, *Chiro-Biz*. It will provide you with a continuing supply of ideas and information, all delivered right to your computer.

I wish you success in reaching and surpassing your goals!

Best wishes,

Ivan

Ivan Delman, DC